How

I Conquered Cancer

A Naturopathic Alternative

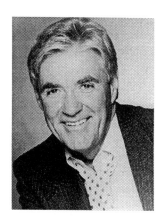

by

Eric Gardiner

International Standard Book Number: 1-885373-11-2 Softcover

Library of Congress Cataloging in Publication Data
Gardiner, Eric 1935 -
How I Conquered Cancer: a naturopathic alternative / by Eric Gardiner.
p. cm.
Includes bibliographical references and index.
ISBN 1-885373-11-2
1. Gardiner, Eric, 1935—Health. 2. Prostate–Cancer-Alternative treatment. 3. Prostate–Cancer–Patients–Colorado–Biography. 4 Naturopathy. I. Title.
RC280.P7G365   1997
362.1'9699463-dc21
[B]   97-21002
                                                 CIP

This book has been prepared to provide accurate and useful information with respect to the subject matter covered. The publisher is not engaged in rendering medical, legal or other professional services. Medical advice should be sought from a competent physician or practitioner. Other expert assistance needed should be sought from the appropriate professional personnel.

While every effort has been made to provide accurate information, the author or publisher cannot be held accountable for errors or omissions. This book is for information purposes only. Neither author or publisher assumes any responsibility for the use or misuse of information contained herein.

For information, call or write:

Emerald Ink Publishing
7141 Office City Dr., Suite 220
Houston, TX 77087-3722
713-643-9945

Printed in the United States of America

Dedication

This book is dedicated to the men of the United States of America. You bought this country piece by piece, from your relatives and friends, from your business associates and agents. You paid for it with your work, skill and daring. You invested your mind and body, your money and your soul, and the only thing you get to take into the shower is your body. That body is under assault from a huge variety of sources, but mostly from you.

This book is dedicated to you because I have a powerful desire for you, the American sons and dads and husbands, not only to have a longer life, but a healthier, happier one. What is the point of living 70, 80 or even more years if those years are hobbled by poor health and the burdens to you and those around you that go with it. So every page is dedicated to you, your prosperity and your good health. You deserve it. YOU are the greatest people on Earth.

Acknowledgements

Authors like to acknowledge a host of people who provide the spark or support or both that help make a book happen. Lou Arrington said "Let's do it," and we did.

Our original plan was to combine our stories into one book, but that changed when she decided she needed more time and detail to tell her story. What you see here is the direct result of her initiative and persistence. The ball has since been given to me and our publisher, Chris Carson, but Lou is the one who started it. It was her decisiveness and support that launched the project. So, to wherever this project goes, we can look back to the launch pad and see the cute little sparkplug brunette from Arizona that lit the fuse.

Thank you Lou.

About the Author

Eric Gardiner attended Northwestern University, Colorado University and the University of Wisconsin where he received his BS majoring in International Economics.

He has traveled all of the contiguous 48 states, western Europe and various intellectual and career territories. He is a nationally rated race car driver in Formula Ford and Sports 2000 cars, a commercial pilot, flight instructor and scuba diver, but his real passion is helping people solve their business and personal problems.

Father of six children, he is an expert in personality profiling and what it means to interpersonal relationships, career choices and stress problems. He co-founded (along with Dr. Sam Houston of the University of Northern Colorado) a company called Sam Houston, Inc. which profiles personalities. Eric has performed over 12,000 personality profiles and has spoken on the subject to audiences large and small all over the country. His insights and creative solutions to interpersonal confrontation and job-related personality conflicts have helped thousands of people find a more peaceful and productive life.

He authored *The Velvet Glove* and *The Velvet Work Glove*. He is completing *The Velvet Workplace*, hiring employees that fit the job like a glove. He founded MotivAward, Inc. an incentive awards company, and Awardcraft, an awards manufacturing company. Now he brings to us his insights into an important condition, prostate cancer, and how it affects people. This condition will afflict most men if they live long enough. He has explained what our parents, teachers, coaches and health professionals have not — how to prevent it, or change it if you have it.

Eighty percent of cancer patients who "survive" this dreaded disease through standard medical treatments later die from it. Standard treatments all too often deal primarily with the symptoms of the disease rather than effecting a cure based on the causes.

This book is a personal testimony to the effectiveness, both healthwise and cost-wise, of naturopathic medical alternatives. Writing in a humorous, entertaining style, Eric Gardiner examines the lifestyle changed he was forced to make after being diagnosed with prostate cancer.

The frank and candid personal evaluation of *standard* versus *naturopathic* approaches and the important information about reducing cancer-causing stress result in a very readable and informative book.

Preface

Not only am I *not* a doctor (M.D. or otherwise), but other than high school and college science courses, I am not at all an authority on cancer. I, perhaps like you, have read scores of articles and books on the subject. I have talked to dozens of people, some of whom are authorities on the subject of health and survival, and cancer in particular. There are literally hundreds if not thousands of books on cancer by authorities and by people who have researched the subject thoroughly, spending years on their projects.

My strength here is my ignorance. I am a frustrated consumer, again perhaps like you. I was brought to the altar of medicine by a society that places medicine and doctors above almost everything else. I was frightened, humiliated, abused and misled. As consumers, you and I have a right to something better. It's our own bodies and our money. By coming at the subject of prostate cancer from your and my side of the fence, I hope to turn on some lights that others have turned on for me. Its a tough path, this life we lead. We need help. Like the old english poem says:

> *"...so let me sit in my house by the side of the road, and be a friend to man."*

I want to extend my hand in help. I know someone will benefit by it. I hope it's you.

Table of Contents

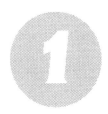

Eric

Christmas is a lousy time of year. The season never seems to live up to the expectations. Was Santa ever really as cheery as the Coca Cola painting? Oh yeah, the tree, the presents, the candy, and the Cancer.

CANCER!

"Yes Mr. Gardiner, there is a growth on your prostate and our biopsy shows it is malignant."

Oh God. What do you do? You sit down and sink low into your chair. You feel the back of your neck begin to sweat and you fell slightly sick to your stomach, maybe more than just slightly. Well, maybe that's not what you would do, but it's what I did. And I cried. Not a lot, but some.

Seven years before (near another Christmas), I had been told I had prostate cancer. I had just taken a physical for my flying license renewal and an old beater doctor with long fingers passed my prostate on his way to my larynx and decided I had cancer. Two days later they called and said "Sorry, it was a mistake. There is no cancer." It seems a blood test had determined I was okay. But I wasn't.

Cancer takes a long time to start in the prostate and it seems Dr. Long Fingers was right and the PSA was wrong. His diagnosis was just slightly premature. There is nothing too surprising here. The year before I was found to have cancer, I decided to take time off my chosen track of good behavior and do some moderate drinking—beer.

I love beer. One is never enough and though I could always pass the driving test, I couldn't pass the belt test. First one belt hole, then another. Soon another coat size and then by "Merry Christmas" I had gained 20 lbs. and .5 point on my PSA. "I think we had better check it," I said.

"I think so," said a new, younger Dr. Long Finger...and the trauma began.

First the T.V. camera—up my rectum. It's not like CBS was trying to buy the rights, but the operator was in there showing me my somewhat enlarged prostate on a T.V. screen. It didn't make the 6 o'clock news, but I'll tell you, it got my attention more than anything I had seen on 60 Minutes. "It doesn't look too bad, but there is a ridge across the top that shouldn't be there. We'll do a series of biopsies and see what they show."

Cancer. That's what it showed. Malignant, downtown, just like millions of other people get, cancer. "Sooner or later all men get prostate cancer," the operator (T.V. man) said. "It's just a matter of time. If you live long enough you'll get it." "And then you'll die from it," were the unsaid words.

It seemed that life had caught up with me. Life had been pretty good to me. Maybe too good. I had good parents that instilled in me: when you want something, you work for it. So I went to work. I won't tell you what my first job was, but it comes out of the back of a chicken, and I shoveled it —for a buck a day. Not bad for an 8 year old kid. By 11, I was economically independent under my parents' roof. I had two paper routes and if I wanted a hamburger or movies I got it, whether anybody liked it or not. High School was work, OK grades and BEER. With my part-time job I delivered it all around the town, including my house. Not to my parents mind you, but to me personally. I bought a car with one week's earnings. I went to college, joined three different fraternities and drank beer. I joined the Air Force, lived in Italy and learned about food. After the Air Force I finished school, got a job and got rich.

Rich enough to have 2 airplanes, 2 houses, 2 horses and steak 5 days a week.

I married a college drop-out who got an F in French but an A+ in bordelaise sauce and bearnaise sauce and, and, and. When I graduated from college I weighed 145 lbs. Two years later I weighed 222. Not bad on my 6'3" skinny frame, but lots and lots of fat, accompanied by martinis and brandy and Chateau LaFitte Rothschild. Isn't that what success was all about: a Lotus in the garage and French wine for dinner.

The divorce started the stress and business problems accelerated it.

One of the causes of cancer is caused by stress and I was getting my Ph.D. We all have our lifetimes full of stress and I was getting mine in two years. More bad business decisions and another bad marriage or two and it was time for bottomsville.

Then I got lucky. I rediscovered some writing and speaking skills and the comeback started. A book, some radio shows, even a couple of 5 watt T.V. shows and my self-worth was starting to come back, but then the year of beer, the prostate exam and cancer. I was going to:

A. Be in pain and die;
B. Get radiated, pee in a bag, get my nuts cut off—and be in pain;
C. Get surgery, pee in a bag, get my nuts cut off—and be in pain...and then die; or
D. None of the above.

I decided "None of the above." The final data isn't in yet, but if you know someone who has prostate cancer (maybe you) and doesn't like A, B, or C—turn the page. You may be able to keep your life, bladder, prostate, money AND your nuts! See you in the next chapter...

The Early Years

Hi, there. I'm the guy in the picture below. The little guy, the one with the patches on his knee, didn't have cancer. He barely had a prostate so how could he have prostate cancer? Well, maybe he did have cancer—at least the beginnings of cancer.

Cancer isn't a bug that jumps out of the air we breathe or from the water we drink. It is a breakdown in our immune system. Like a car, a problem can exist in the brakes or drive train or engine. We know that something isn't working right. The car won't start or run, or it won't stop. There is a problem and it almost surely didn't start when you found the problem. A flat tire is perhaps different, but even a flat tire could come from a puncture that you got miles or weeks before.

My prostate cancer was caused by my big brother Robert. You can see the beautiful leather boots that I am wearing in the picture with the duckling in the pond. I loved those boots. They were my

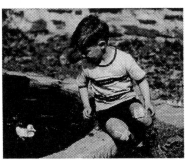

pride and joy. Putting them on made me feel good, big, powerful, run-through-anything powerful. I could climb big trees, jump ditches, even swing on the big kids' "Devil Swing" in those boots. They didn't have a pocket for a penknife like boots have today but they fit, they were mine and I loved them.

My brother decided that he would make a sling-shot. He found just the right piece of Y-shaped wood. He found an old rubber innertube for the sling part. He needed something to form the pocket for the stone he would shoot. He searched far and wide before he decided that he needed a piece of my leather boots for his slingshot. One day I went to put on my prized possessions, my pride and joy, and a big chunk was missing out of one of them.

I was crushed. Not only was my brother four years older, he was much bigger and stronger. Revenge was out of the question. My boots were ruined—gone for good.

How about a new pair from my parents? This was 1939. The Depression was just winding down and new boots were not to be. How about an apology from my brother? Something like "I'm sorry." It was not forthcoming. How about sympathy or a sign of caring, love or understanding from my parents—anybody? No.

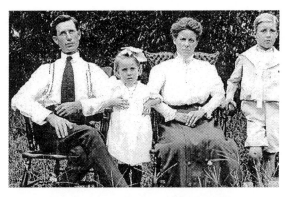

My grandfather, Aunt Blanche, grandmother and father. My grandfather was a brilliant hard-nosed stick-in-the-mud with no flair for business. My father was a bright guy with a flair for music, acting and pool. He met my mother (an older woman) in amateur theatre and they bred five more performers.

Unresolved conflict appears on almost every list of causes of cancer I've seen. How many men could tell similar stories? Probably more than not.

A few years later, my sister Virginia was angry with me about something and grabbed my toy airplane I was playing with. This was 1944 and radio shows like Jack Armstrong, Sky King and Hop Harrigan filled the minds of most young boys. All the 60 year-old guys remember. You spread your arms like airplane wings and ran around having mock airplane fights with your buddies. If you had only a few toys, that concentrated their individual value. If you spent a lot of time with them, that increased their value further. I spent a lot of time. I had one toy, my wooden airplane. As I was pleading for her not to, she broke off the wings and tail and then threw it on the ground. She was six years older than I was. She was bigger and stronger. Revenge would have been futile. I had no support system. My mother was busy with other things. My father was overseas killing Germans.

Does this stuff cause cancer? Maybe. Probably. Yes. Enough unresolved conflict is *at least* a contributor to prostate cancer.

Yeah, but boots, model airplanes, how about polio and world hunger and war and appendicitis and AIDS and heart disease? Yes, those are bigger issues. They are more important. But this is me. This is my prostate. This is my cancer, and this is why—partly.

If I was going to beat this thing and keep it beat, I had to know where it came from and how to treat not just my prostate but also my head and my memories.

So cancer comes not just from what I put and keep in my mind but also what I put in my stomach. Boy, did I (put it in my stomach)!

So drink: chug-a-lug, chug-a-lug, chug-a-lug. Now drink: chug a lug, on through the night. My first year at The University of Wisconsin, and if I was going to be a good Chi Phi pledge, I had to know how to drink, throw up and drink some more. It also helps to know how to clean up...puke that is, because that is part of a job as a good Chi Phi Fraternity pledge. My parents put me on a great path: go to school, be part of ROTC, graduate, fly airplanes in Korea, and if I didn't get killed or stuck in a POW camp, I could get out in 20 years as a Colonel. Or I could resign after 7 years and go to work for a Fortune 500 Company and have a family. Kind of like being a POW, if you know what I mean.

To Hell with that idea...I'm going to leave Wisconsin, go to Northwestern and study acting. Mrs. Fisher gave me a F in "Voice and Diction." My voice and diction were all right (I was one of few that I know of in the class that actually made money in the media) but she had this deranged idea that I should go to class. What a novel idea, but I was too busy selling Electrolux vacuum cleaners to pay for school and my commitment to the Theta Zi fraternity, to keep up my end of the bargain of keeping Theta Zi the best animal house on campus.

My grades weren't good but I got A's in party. One of the sororities had a beautiful tie and coat, purple passion party at a fine Chicago Hotel.

The band made the mistake of taking a "break" and when they returned the party-goers were dueling with their instruments. Using the trumpets and trombones as if they were swords. Clarinets were being used to bang on drums and drumsticks were used to beat the hell out of the tuba. And there was our fraternity brother, an all-American fullback dancing on the table with his pants slowly descending. Wait a minute. Isn't he supposed to be in Baton Rouge playing football the next day? Well, LSU will have to wait. This was before the days of DUI and points so it was assumed every student got drunk every weekend, unless your father had a lot of money. In that case, you got drunk every night.

The animal house got out of anyone's control. Three presidents were impeached, the kitchen was assaulted every night and the University made us take down our homecoming decoration, something about it being lewd and insulting. I helped design it and I can tell you it was wonderful. By today's standards, it was tame.

Because Evanston was dry, we rented "Halls" outside of the city limits and drank several toasts to the Women's Christian Temperance Union. Their international headquarters were in Evanston, Illinois in 1955. At one of our parties the empty cans were stacked so high we had to stand on a ladder to keep them going higher. Of course someone fell off the ladder into the cans, but that noise was overshadowed by a louder crash of the 400 lb. safe falling through the ground floor to the basement. It seems the brothers found it on the 4th floor and decided a good way to get it open was to throw it down the stairwell.

Greasy breakfasts, sweet lunches and fat-filled dinners were filling my system with every kind of blockage. The beer was doing a number on my liver and kidneys and less than 8 hours per night of sleep was slowly reducing my immune system to less than its intended efficiency.

"If you're going to hear the tune, you have to pay the piper" was 100 years away. After my sophomore year, I decided to be a flyboy. The Air Force decided I would make a great paperpusher. They gave me a test and it showed I would be good at making sure targets for our bombers had the exact and correct target number identification. The numbers were about 12 inches and 100 digits long, and I can tell you none of mine were right. It was like putting a blind man in charge of the bombsight. Fortunately none of "my" bombs were dropped, thereby saving hundreds of cows, streams, and small roads from utter destruction. Enemy airfields, critical bridges, and railroad marshaling yards would have remained untouched.

In 1958 I was paid $85.00 a month by your government to live on a base in Germany and drink all the beer Germany could make. A full liter of German beer was less than 25 cents. Me and several friends tried, but it wasn't even close. Germany won. They could make it faster than we could drink it. We were also given the mission of protecting the U.S. shores from the attacks of the European women. As far as I know we won that one. A few might have slipped through as wives, but most are still over there. But there was a catch. We had to buy them beer or they would invade. It was tough but...well you know.

Beer, bratwursts, I'm sure my little prostate was starting to have ideas even then. In Italy it was spaghetti, red wine, salad, Buton brandy and cow stomach. Plenty of cheese, fat-filled Genoa salami and, oh yes, the Chow Hall kept up the supply of things to coat my intestines, my arteries and feed the parasites. Guess I didn't mention those unfriendly little rascals. Some people would tell you that not only does cancer thrive on parasites, it depends on them. More on that later.

This was a hill climb race car that I bought for $200 in 1958 and sold it for $200 a few months later. Clean models today sell for hundreds of thousands of dollars. Am I smart or what? This one had an aluminum body and a 2 liter Bristol engine, one of the fastest accelerating cars I ever drove. Not bad for a public servant earning $86 a month.

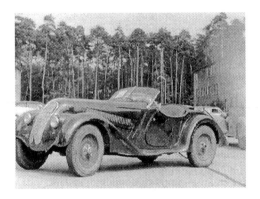

The U.S. Air Force in Europe in 1957 was the worst and the best. On the one hand, I had a job for which I was totally unsuited. On the other hand, almost every G.I. was a prized target for every European mother. Remember the WWII quote from England about the G.I. station there?

"They're overpaid, over-sexed and over here."

Twelve years later, it was all still true. Virtually everywhere I went, I was welcomed, especially by Mama. So in the daytime, I had this idiotic job working for 'career' officers and enlisted men who for the most part couldn't make it on the outside. They lorded it over guys like me who had a choice of signing up or being drafted. I met a few notable exceptions, a black General, B. O. Davis, being one of them. But the majority of my bosses were "in for twenty" and were hanging on for dear life. It was either "Shut up and do your job" or "Go to jail." Kinda puts a stress on one's work situation.

After work, we went on the town and we were treated so good it ruined us forever. It was as if we were all Hollywood stars. I traveled a lot and everywhere I went—from Oslo, Norway to Rome—I was graciously and warmly welcomed. Compare that with what G.I.s in the states were treated like in the late 50's: underpaid, overworked and "not with my daughter!"

So there I was in a stress-filled stupid job in the daytime and hero worship at nights, weekends and those great, long military leaves, 30 days a year. Does this cause cancer? Does worry and emotional whiplash cause cancer? Does it *start* to break down the immune system? In combination with all the other stuff I was doing to my system the answer apparently was—yes.

In 1958 I was transferred from Ramstein, Germany to Aviano, Italy. People who know both would tell you I went from a bad place to a good place. Well, kind of.

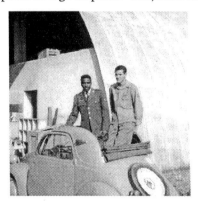

I went from working for 25 mostly losers to 1 total imbecile. He was responsible for my life and yet he had no idea of what I did or how I did it. He was a foul-mouthed, ugly, stupid, obnoxious slob who made three times as much money as I did and could send me to jail in a finger-snap if he didn't like me or what I was doing. He had six stripes; I had one. His boss, a major, had only one reason for being a major. He spoke Czechoslovakian. We didn't use the language. We didn't need the language (after 1945) and here was this guy trying to do something with absolutely nothing in the world to do.

The major decided I couldn't have a Christmas leave because the "Unit" was screwed up. When I pointed out that my section was not only not screwed up but in great shape, the major said it's too bad. If some can't go, none can go. I said I might be there but I wouldn't do anything. That was the wrong thing to say. He beat a huffy exit. When I heard the words "court martial him" come from the other room, I realized I not only wasn't going to have my Christmas in Copenhagen with friends, I might have the Christmas turkey in jail. A public apology was given—believe me it was sincere and shortly thereafter I got a promotion.

My job in part was to order "Secret" target maps to have for our pilots to find their way to their assigned targets, airfields, bridges, etc. I would order twenty-five copies of a given map, and quick as a wink, a month later I would get two hundred and fifty. I didn't want two hundred and fifty. I didn't need two hundred and fifty. The taxpayers didn't want to pay for two hundred and fifty but that was the drill. So I had a high-tech disposable method. I burned them, one at a time, in a fifty-five gallon drum. But don't worry. You were protected from secret agents who would come and take them from me. I was provided with a side arm (a .45 caliber pistol) with which to fend off such an attack. I was prepared to defend the security of the United States. There was one small problem. I was not allowed to have any bullets. I don't know why.

So here I was, doing this great work for people, none of whom had a 100 I.Q. and was under great pressure to do one thing I was really not good at. Behave. And the consequences were jail if I didn't.

Sixty miles away was a place on the Adriatic called Lignano Sabbiadorro (of the Golden Sand). On any given weekend, there were many hundreds, if not thousands, of single ladies from England, Austria, Germany and other places, whose fondest hope was to meet and romance and if possible marry a young American. And the price was right.

A hotel room was eighty-four CENTS. A good meal ran the same. There was no way one could drink a dollar's worth of wine, all from an income of $150 per month with room and board free.

I had the great good fortune to meet a lovely young lady who was on the Austrian ski team, quite a feat in 1958 or '59. On meeting her mother, I and my friends were warmly invited to their home in Graz, Austria. A month later, my four buddies and I arrived at 2 in the morning after a long drive. The table was set with all the beer, wurst and goodies we could consume. Over the weekend, we were given the grand tour of the city and evirons and treated generally like much admired and appreciated young men. The answer to your question is "Yes," and it was wonderful. This situation was not the exception or even routine. It was the rule.

Question: Does this emotional whipsaw cause prostate cancer?

Answer: Sooner or later—maybe.

So out of the service I go. Europe is saved, now it's time to finish school. But wait a minute...is booze and greasy food the only thing that causes cancer? How about a guilt trip or two, or two thousand? Remember the sixth commandment. That baby caught up to me two years after most people. I was 16 when "it" happened. God did that feel good. Oh Oh. No that's for married folks and to even THINK about carnal knowledge is a mortal sin. Even liking the IDEA of being sexually aroused is a sure trip to Hades. So when the urge that procreates the world came calling I went into an immediate and continuous guilt trip. The good folks at Saint Monica's laid such a heavy fear on me that "that" stress started in spades and it laid open the doors to fear and guilt and anger and THAT causes cancer.

In the ideal family, a support group helps us learn right from wrong. There is a balance in learning these lessons with discipline on one side and love on the other. Think of it as the stick and the carrot with love and affection added onto both the stick and the carrot. Positive self-image comes from the success side of the equation. The most successful coaches, the most successful teachers, the most successful parents achieve their ends by showing their players, students and children the way to do something and then praise success while lovingly criticizing failure.

The stick alone will work with animals and with people, but we know now that people and animals do better with love and praise. It's faster, cheaper and more effective—there's one problem, however. If the coach, teacher or parents have a self-image problem, the chances of a balanced learning situation is at least low. It seems incredible to me that so many people can go through school, grow up and be successful people and still think deep down that they are really not very good, worthwhile or deserving of happiness.

I've gone to enough 'help' groups to believe that half the country is in a poor self-worth stew and the other half doesn't care. A book, *The Codependency Conspiracy,* points out that over 85% of the people who go through self-help groups eventually solve their own problems. The others stay in the cycle or pay to get fixed.

When we feel good about ourselves, usually there is a good person somewhere behind. All it takes is one—one someone— who believes in you, who trusts you, who praises you.

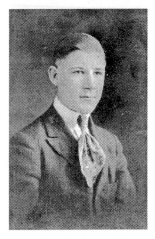

Is this guy a stud or what? My father in college. Kept his wife and his prostate. He died in the saddle—giving a speech at age 77.

Praise was a rare commodity when I was growing up. All of us are too "something." I was too thin. I was six feet three inches tall and weighed 145 pounds. I had fly-away hair that no amount of Brylcreem™ could keep presentable for more than five minutes. I had no whiskers (I didn't shave regularly until I was about twenty-five) and no body hair. What a mess. Besides, I had an above-average amount of pimples.

The lucky ones had a parent or someone who told you, as Barry Manilow says, "You're not so bad." I didn't. Or if I did, I couldn't hear them. Because of this lousy self-image, I made poor choices, bad decisions. I had not found my inner voice yet so I had no guide resource.

My parents had led an exemplary life and were very successful in their marriage and life course.

I was all alone and doing poorly. Without a loving guidance and support system, life was one stressful situation after another. The young bodies can take it but there comes a time when the stresses add up. If the "can-do" self-confidence, self-worth isn't there, the body starts to give up. Somewhere in the system, something starts to break down. In the American man, it is frequently the prostate.

The authorities know and tell us that cancer is caused by a whole bunch of stuff— what you eat, drink, breathe, think and more.

To get rid of it, you have to change all of this. If someone had just told me when I

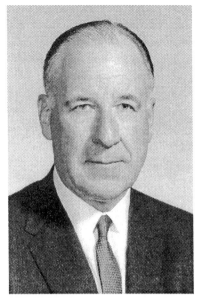

My father at retirement, age 70. He wrote prolifically: safety and training materials. For his work at D-Day in Normandy and WWII, he received the Croix de Guerre and the bronze star.

He retired as a Bird Colonel. Most of his business associates called him Colonel.

was 20 or 30 or even 40, that I was riding on a path to sure pain and poverty, then I would have changed. That's what we're here for, to tell you, so you can change. Sure, antacids stop the stomach upset but they don't stop the cause. If you knew that you were going to get cancer from your current lifestyle, Tums™ and Valium™ notwithstanding—would you change? Of course you would, especially if the changes you would make would be pleasurable and inexpensive, probably costing you even less than your spending now.

But I'm getting ahead of myself. Let me continue to show you how getting cancer was almost a sure thing and how conquering it was going against the tide.

Did you know that you can buy a cheap roast, cover it with mustard to tenderize it, then burn it on the grill, and if you get the college coed drunk enough on cheap beer she will half-believe she's getting steak.

Well, that was the drill. With the beautiful "Flat Irons" at the University of Colorado as a back-drop we burned dozens of blade

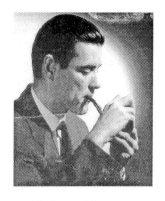

My first modeling picture. They even paid me. I think it was $25 an hour.

roast "steaks" and drank dozens of cases of homemade beer and pleased the evenings of many a beautiful lady, hard on their way to finding out what real consumption means.

My drive time radio show on the local AM station made me a legend in my own time so companionship was frequent if not con-stant. Of course, the guilt trip was a burden and those magic words every hop-to-it college guy loves to hear "I'm pregnant" added a few more layers of guilt and stress. How that all worked out is another story, but it did teach me how to become a profes-sional-quality worrier.

Somehow I managed to get through school (partly because of another sister) and got a great job offer. Back in the early 60's there were more jobs than people so we all got good job offers.

I thickened the plot a little bit by arranging to hear those magic words "I'm pregnant" again, so before I was even out of college I had a family and was married to a teenager who made the world's best Hollandaise sauce. I put on 70 pounds of pure fat in two years. I also met the local beer wholesaler and thanks to a knowledgeable brother-in-law, got the pressure tanks, etc. to have my own beer on tap for only a dollar a gallon. Thanks to mutual meals, my wife and I both became blobs. My exercise pro gram consisted of riding the riding lawn mower and my wife's work-out consisted of beating the Hollandaise sauce, sometimes even twice when it curdled, which it did frequently.

We both were ex-Catholics, so the religion of guilt was replaced with...nothing. Most people are born into some kind of religious affinity and for many people it serves them well. It is amazing to look in the Yellow Pages and see just how many choices there are. While not up to the numbers of lawyers, churches make up scores or hundreds of choices in most metro areas. So why all the cancer? I had friends who had as many problems as I did and they put on the Sunday suit and went to hear the sermon. Interaction with them showed me two things: they thought their brand was the only way to the promised land and they weren't doing any better at being friendly and more caring than anybody else.

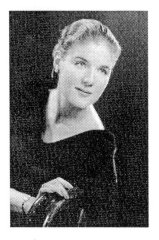

This is my sister Patricia shortly after she graduated from the University of Wisconsin. She and her her husband had eight restaurants and a 10,000 square foot home on Chicago's North Shore. We all worked hard and did well. No divorce. Four kids. A+.

Still, like most people, I was searching for an answer, a guide, a coach. The idea of having to go through an intermediary left me cold. Why did I need somebody or some institution between me and my *source*? I tried that as a Catholic for twenty years and it produced guilt-wrapped answers. I knew lots of people but none that I knew had answers that I believed in or trusted. I had had a *religious* upbringing but not a *spiritual* one.

We all have a spiritual side or resource and when we choose to dump it, we need a substitute. I choose Heilemans Old Style™, ribeye steak and antacids; asparagus Hollandaise, baked potato

17

with sour cream and lots of butter and antacids. And for dessert, Old Style™ and antacids.

It is hard to know how much stress we put on our minds or bodies when we deny them what they need. In retrospect, I would guess that the body is very much tied to its *invisible* resources. Science is coming to the powerful conclusion that the unseen healers are in many cases more powerful than regular *Mediums*. Recent studies show a powerful statistical benefit of prayers, both first and third party. Just praying for someone helps them get well. When we pray for ourselves, it has a powerful impact.

At this time, I was more into *goal setting* and *management by objectives*. They worked and my world expanded.

The gods of business were quite good so fine wines lobster and stronger beverages were added to the menu. We were really climbing the mountain.

While digging the shallow hole for the 18 foot excuse for a swimming pool, I turned bright red almost like Santa from the waist up. I let my belt out a notch and forgot about it. Your government decided I needed a new G.I. bill. Since I had finished school on my own, I took advantage of their "commercial flying" program.

The unknown benefit of this was the biannual physical. That was the avenue to the uncovering of the "C" word. Flying is not what you would call a cardiovascular activity. It is mostly sitting and doing nothing. How about skiing? That would be a good workout. We lived near Chicago.

I am second from the right. This was my first twin engine airplane.

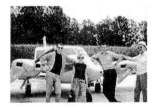

Life was going great. Let's see— was that 8 or 10 steaks a week?

There were two major choices. Drive for 1½ hours to Alpine Mountain (mountains are now 200 feet high), wait in line for 45 minutes and ski down the hill for 45 seconds—slowly. Not exactly a workout.

Choice Two was to drive 7 hours to upper Michigan. There was no long line because anything longer than 10 minutes standing still meant sure death. One could encounter 50-60 MPH wind speeds while standing still at the top of the hill. A 6 hour ski day consisted of 2 hours of icy skiing, 2 hours of the "death wait" in line and 2 hours of recovering in the lodge.

So if not flying or skiing, what could I do for an exercise program? I bought a ski machine and damaged all of the furniture within falling distance. The machine had giant rubber bands that if used just right could propel a user through a 2¼" pine door. So my weight hung around 220, my suit size settled at 44XL and my frustrations at looking at my mirror turned me into a nightmare. I tried a couple of diets, including liquid protein, truly a potion that could cause maggots to throw up. Dr. Atkins did no better for me than most. How about the water diet? The toilets got exercised, I got angry.

Life became a blur of wine, food and not much fun. My Gelucil™ antacid bill started running into hundreds of dollars a year. People could hear me coming because my gelusil packages rattled.

I had them in one pocket or another at all times. And I frequently had a white ring around my mouth, not from milk, but Gelusil.™

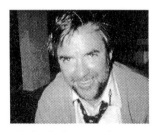

1985. Drinking is fun, right? It makes us handsome and charming. Not! I tried to keep up drinking with my German friends. They seemed to be OK. I got stupid and went to sleep. Everyone who drinks should have a picture of themselves when they are "overserved." It makes stopping easier. How do you think this affected my prostate?

Something had to give, it was me. I don't know who mentioned divorce first, but our fifteen year marriage was over faster than you can eat a Tums™ tablet. We split it right down the middle. She got the house, car, kids, bank accounts, furniture, insurance, cash, jewelry, friends etc., and I got 3 bookcases and a convertible couch that the cat had pissed on. Oh, I did get to keep the business and a child support payment that enabled her and her new boyfriend to live quite nicely.

Have you heard of night sweats? I was the Niagara Falls of night sweats.

Fate was kind enough to provide me with companionship fairly soon, but they had to wear rubber suits because I sweat. I was just worried sick and frightened to death. No nice house, no airplane, no bank account, no furniture, no nothing, and then those national debt child support payments, now that will cause you worry. But if you miss one, then it's jail time. Now, that will give you the sweats. I didn't know it then, but on reflection it was probably then that my prostate started to dance.

It is hard to tell someone who has not done it how painful and stressful divorce with children is. The media have done a good job portraying the sad state of affairs for the mother and children. The movie Kramer vs. Kramer gave some insights into the plight of the father, but it is the non-custodial father (which I was) that is so awful. I was allowed every other weekend with the children. I'm sure you know the routine. There was one catch. They wouldn't come. I would drive up to the house and the children would appear at the window, then disappear. They wouldn't come out. I would drive away...alone.[1]

Somehow I kept my life together and after facing the big 'B' I was able to avoid bankruptcy and go on to new prosperity.

The best thing to do when you get through a divorce is to go find a tall beautiful brunette who had a terrible relationship with her father and who subsequently hated men. Besides, there are no morality problems because sex has a low priority, coming somewhere after craft lessons and feeding her giant cat "Tramp." I won't bother you with the details but what was left from the first

---

1. It seems the mother and her new boyfriend had told them they didn't have to go. And if they wouldn't, there would be special treats and treatment. This is one very effective way at "getting back" at the non-custodial parent. It isn't very fun. It isn't legal, but it does work. The youngest, Laura, who did come at first, was ridiculed and put down. Soon, even she stopped coming. Like I said, it works. The children, now grown, are still paying the price.

marriage was lost in the second. I did learn that a good way to reduce stress is to run. So I ran up the mountain, down the mountain and around the mountain house. I had bought a lovely home in the mountains west of Denver.

I hired a friend of my new wife to run the business. Soon, my wife (who became my ex-wife) and her friend and our child (yeah, we had one, am I cool or what?) and my business were all pretty well gone. I took a stab at a few dozen more relationships and then God came and said "don't do that any more." Yeah, I found the Big Guy.

My pendulum swings with Religion-God-Spirituality had gone from total fear when I was a young child and a student at a Catholic school to a form of atheism with a slow-growing awareness that God wasn't responsible for my problems. I was. As a young child, I was immersed in the pageantry of it all. My vivid imagination allowed me to feel the fires of Hell and "know" that I would burn there if I didn't obey the rules. With puberty, the rules ran headlong into nature. Everyday became an exercise in guilt and shame. Even innocent dates became cesspools of urge and shame, urge and shame. At a beach party after my senior year in high school, I touched my first breast as an adult and felt compelled to attend Mass every day for six weeks to assuage my guilt.

The message was not "Be smart. Be in control of yourself. Wait until you are in a financially secure and socially acceptable place to express yourself sexually." The message was "This is wrong and if you do it or even think about it, you are bad and evil and you will go to Hell." The good news was that I didn't have any children during my teens and early twenties. The bad news was that I lived a life filled with frustration and guilt. God became this heartless, hurtful, frustrating person who gave me urges with no resolution, imagination with no fulfillment, and a need for love but with "Danger: Keep Out!" signs.

Finally, I met a fellow student in college who showed me the folly of my guilt-ridden thinking. God became a distant force. Guilt disappeared and pregnancy shortly followed. My student friend was not there to help me with the consequences.

Over the years, God was referred to in the self-help books I was reading as a powerful private presence in our lives. The more I tried of their technique of getting in touch with this resource, the more I felt a bond growing. The more I listened to others who lived their religion within a system or regimen, the more it sounded phony, unreal and contrived. The people I most respected were those who had their own relationship with their own God. They seemed most at peace. That's what I wanted—peace.

On the night of December 23rd, 1989, I stood on my porch asking for answers.

The snow-capped peaks of the continental divide glistened in the moonlight. The night was dead still. I looked around me at the majestic 300 year-old trees standing as they had through fire, pestilence and storm. I wanted peace and purpose in my fragmented, troubled and stress-filled life.

"Lord, what am I here for?" I called out.

I looked down at the ground eight feet below the porch and saw my moonlit shadow. A gentle awareness asked me, "Do you want to be yourself or the shadow of yourself?"

Suddenly, a strong wind came up. The tall evergreens started bending in its wake and I heard a rustling of paper down below on the ground. The wind died down but I still heard the rustling and rattling of this paper blowing around below me. I walked down the stairs and picked up this section of the Denver paper that had been blowing around. I didn't remember any paper ever blowing around the house before, but this one was. It contained the obituary section. I felt moved to pick it up and look inside. It contained the obituary of a man I knew in Denver. He had died on December 19th—my birthday—of cancer.

Had I been visited by a higher power? I called a friend named Sam Houston. He and his wife drove sixty miles to see me. We sat in my living room conversation pit and talked about it. He was a friend, confidant and business associate. He thought I had been visited by a higher power. We reviewed the incident. Sam was a part-time priest and had administered the last rites to our friend who died on my birthday: Had I been visited by a higher power? I thought so then. I think so now. I still have the newspaper. It is in a collector's "Eagle" box, a limited production 4x8x2 box that I had bought one year before, whose production number is 023. The night I found the paper was 12/23.

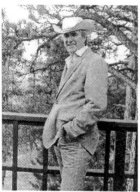

That was the beginning of a stronger relationship with what I call my guide. It (he, she) has never guided me to be mean or hurtful or vengeful. It has never been purposeless or aimless and its guidance has never been wrong. I have tried hard to seek its advice. At first, I used it once or twice a month and it took me days more to get an answer. Now I use it hundreds of times a day and I get my answers in micro seconds.

The rattling newspaper grabbed my attention. Yeah, He was there!

Late one cold winter night I had walked out on the porch of my 4600 sq.ft. home and said "Please, God, help me get out of here." Eight months later I was gone.

In the meantime, I got a call from my brother from Purgatory (something is always wrong) who said I was going to die. (I told you something was always wrong). It seems he had *Hemocromotosis*, and therefore so must I. So I should go find out. I got my bi-annual flight physical. They also checked for hemocromatosis and concluded I had it. They gave me the name of a specialist who said he could see me in two weeks. I said I'll be right over. Yes, I had it, a liver biopsy would show how far it had progressed. The next day they did the biopsy—a two hour slight inconvenience that went wrong.

PAIN? You talk about pain? He missed with his little biopsy tool, hit my bile duct and I felt pain!

My house had just sold. I had hemocromotosis and I was trying to hit the road to I knew not where. Three days later I left the hospital (no, not two hours of inconvenience), had Thanksgiving with a friend and started bleeding all over the Western United

States. That's how you treat hemocromotosis, give blood, or dump it. I was feeling kind of good. My brother was wrong. I was not going to die from overly iron rich blood (hemocromotosis). They had caught it in plenty of time. All I had to do was give blood for the rest of my life and things would be O.K. If I didn't donate, I would die of heart or liver disease or such. The next few years were spent traveling and doing business across the country. I visited the 48 contiguous states and had generally a good time. I did enough business to pay my way, saw the country and ate at the best the Denny's and McDonald's had to offer. No relationships. No alcohol. I learned to live alone. Occasionally I would visit friends that would keep me around for a while, but mostly I was on consulting assignments with lodging provided, or I was motel man. I figured I stayed at over two hundred different Motel 6's west of the Mississippi alone.

I got my blood tested every year. Iron was O.K, PSA was slightly over 5.

I met some people in Kansas who wanted me to market their mineral pills. I did. I took them myself. My PSA went down. My dental health improved. My energy went up. I skied better and stronger than I had in 20 years. My PSA went to the high 4's. I missed having a house, family and a relationship but the freedom was great. If I didn't like where I was or who I was with—I left. Neat.

A friend I met while skiing, asked me to help him and his wife straighten a few marital wrinkles. By this time I was a published author, had done several T.V. and radio shows about using profiles to make one's 5 lives (business, financial, personal, health & spiritual) better and people were willing to pay me to help them find better suited employees. The system worked and I did to. I had established a growing bond with my higher power. I was making right decisions and not making wrong ones. In early March of 1994, after a grueling trip to & through New York to see my friend with the relationship problems, I ask my "Guide" if it was OK to have a couple of beers. My guide said "yes." The beer tasted great.

My friends wife said "leave." A year of beer later my PSA was 5.7 and the doctor said Cancer.

At first I felt betrayed by my "guide" for letting me drink beer and get cancer. Now I have a different view. As you will see, it had what I trust was a higher purpose. Come on along, I'll show you why I feel that way.

The Coming

When does cancer begin?

I don't know—probably when we're born.

Let me emphasize I am no cancer expert. I'm just a guy like you, who was told he had cancer, and if you haven't been told you have a fatal disease, you just can't imagine the feeling. Yeah, we've all been scared in wrecks or injuries or near misses, but cancer...it's different, and worse. I'm told there are six or seven different kinds of things that contribute to the disease. It's almost surely not a bug that we get that grows and makes a growth and thus we die.

The modern world has brought us so many wonderful things. We have had quantum leaps each decade or less in science, mathematics, chemistry and yes, medicine. Unfortunately we have done major damage to our food chain. Most of us eat everyday and what we are eating is killing us. The air is bad. Workplace conditions have air that goes from stale to outright poison. As we have improved the insulation and air penetration of our homes they have become carcinogen boxes that are filled with the air from all of the chemicals that we store there.

The water that we drank in 1776 was almost surely polluted near town but mountain streams were probably okay. Today the earth shows pollution from pole to pole. Virtually everywhere has air, water and therefore land pollution. Some of our bodies can handle it. Some can't. As the population and pollution grows, more and more of us won't be able to handle it and the problem will grow—fast.

In the meantime there is a lot we do to bring on the diseases we have.

1. We eat inappropriate foods.
2. We drink inappropriate beverages.
3. We don't exercise.
4. We inherit "weak" genes.
5. We catch "germs" that our immune system can't handle—in

part because of 1, 2 or 3 above.

6. We choose to live in a hassled environment.

7. We worry ourselves sick.

Because I had lived less than a pristine life, I was not 100% surprised when an FAA flight physical examiner said I had cancer. That was in 1988. It was a great shock but frankly, I didn't believe him because I didn't like him. This was a one hour exam to renew my pilots license and I had no idea how they came to that conclusion, something about a blood test. Two days later they called and said it had been a mistake, that I was okay. My pilots license medical was approved and I went on my way. No one said anything so I didn't do anything.

Most men who are diagnosed with prostate cancer work. They have a career whether it is flying airliners, working at a desk, a computer, a machine, driving a tractor, whatever. Most of them are unhappy. I see conflicting data that says most people are happy — I think most are unhappy.[1] Most people are unhappy for the simple reason that they are square pegs in round holes. You've heard of the Peter Principle that says people rise to their level of incompetence. That logic goes hand in hand with the philosophy that says "We hire from within." By reducing the labor pool to those already on board, you create a greater chance of engaging the Peter Principle.

There is stress in a frustrating job. Unless you have one of those miracle twenty minute commutes, there is also stress in getting to and from work. Is it any wonder that we see tremendous increases in the use of stress reducers such as prescriptions and illicit drugs? Booze is making it to television along with beer and wine. How many people join Bally's and other exercise parlors around the country to get rid of stress? The sad part is—for most people, it isn't working. *"100% of men will get prostate cancer. It's*

---

1. I do computerized personality profiling. We use the results to hire people and find better job/person relationships. It is not time for a commercial but the stuff works. We clearly show job person relationships and are able to quantify them.

just a question of time." So said the medical technician who worked for Dr. Goodblood (not his real name).

In the last ten years, businesses have practiced "sharpening their pencils," "leaning down," and scaring the hell out of everybody without a Golden Parachute (which is almost everybody). Labor—from executives on down to the newest timecard puncher—has been reduced to a commodity, like a gallon of gas or a pound of meat. There is almost no loyalty from company to worker, or worker to company. Sure, there are exceptions, but they just make the rule that much more clear. I was fired from my first job out of college. The new manager wanted to make a name for himself. Because I had been hired by the president of this major corporation, this would be a good way to show his power. No interview, no excuse, just "You're fired." They said something about driving too fast. Not a bad trait, I figured, for a new sales rep. I suppose I should have slowed down when my boss was riding with me. I should have gotten my clue when he threw up the second time. Just kidding.

So I went and told my wife who was pregnant and she shortly went into labor. We were going to name the child "Asshole" after my ex-boss, but that was a boy's name and we had a girl.

The stress of being fired with a first child on the way pales in comparison to what many of the "outplaced" people experience today. I did a seminar for a group called *Forty Plus* in Denver. There were over a hundred (mostly men) who were over forty years old, out of a job, looking at bills for house, food, clothes, insurance and the like. How ghastly. Most were not marketing types. They had no real skills in selling themselves and "were off-the-tree ripe" for scam artists who were going to help them find a job. The horror stories are rampant and the prostate cancer rolls on.

So between job stress and family stress and self-abuse, I was doing what many men do: I was cooking my immune system. Sooner or later, something was going to give. I had gotten away with it so far. Everything checked out, if not normal, at least okay.

December of '95 was different. I knew things were not right. I had gained weight, and I had been "bad with beverages." As usual I went in for my iron blood test that included a PSA measurement. Three days later I called for the data and they told me the iron numbers were good but that my PSA had registered 5.5. The year before it had been 4.7. I was worried. I called Dr. Goodblood, the urologist I had used over the last few years. I disliked him personally. He was aloof and cold. At a previous appointment, he left before seeing me and without even saying anything. His nurse came in to tell me that he was called away for an emergency. Couldn't he even stick his neck in to say he was sorry?

Anyway, I went to see him again in early January 1996. Rubber gloves, slime juice and in she goes, only this time he had an enlarged target. My prostate had grown from 35 centimeters to 45 centimeters, *not* a good place to put on weight. There was a helpful technician there with his own set of gloves and slime juice. He pointed out that sooner or later all of "us guys were going to get it." He had this mini TV camera on the end of a probe. He slipped it in and I didn't feel a thing. By this time my anus was so greased up they could have put the "Queen Mary" up there and I wouldn't have known. Anyway the TV camera did its job and I could see everything.

It was really neat as he moved the probe (camera) around. I could see my prostate. Yep, it was about the size of a walnut. It had a "ridge" along its length that he said wasn't supposed to be there. He probed around as I watched the little TV Medicine truly is amazing. He looked around at some other organ which seemed to be okay. He said that the prostate was slightly enlarged and there was that "ridge."

Dr. Goodblood came in and took an extended look. He asked if I had trouble urinating.

"Not really," I said, "but it does seem a little slower."

"How about at night time? Do your have to go to the bathroom a lot?"

"Not really. Perhaps a little more, once in awhile, but there's not really much change."

He discussed the ridge that wasn't supposed to be there but was. He said he wanted to take six samples of my prostate to test for malignancy. At the previous office visit, I had signed a consent form so he was ready to go. He put six little x's on the TV screen that showed me where the biopsy would be taken. They made an angular pattern that went across the ridge from left to right.

He left the room and came back with a probe that looked like a grabber you would use to reach down through a sewer grate to fetch your lost coin or ring. This grabber was not three feet long but it looked too long to me.

What was I supposed to say? "I don't really want you to do this"? Perhaps this is what a woman feels like when she is exposed to intercourse the first time. Well, I didn't really want to do it, but it was too late.

He inserted the grabber. I could see it going in much further than I assumed was healthy. He said this would probably sting. STING? Well, it really wasn't that bad—kind of like a dentist pulling on your tooth before the novocaine has completely taken effect.

"How are you doing?" he asked.

I braved up and mumbled something like "okay."

Five more stings and he was through. He gave me a paper to read that said I might bleed, but not to worry. Right! He gave (not really—this is a misuse of the language—they don't give you anything) me some medicine and said the only real concern was if my temperature should rise. Sex would be okay but maybe bloody. Talk about role reversal! It might be better to wait a few days.

"Sorry, honey. I can't tonight. It's that time and I might ruin the sheets."

He was right. When I first urinated and had a bowel movement, things were bright red. Bright red! A few days later, everything settled down, but my ejaculate stayed a little red for a few weeks. I was going to have to decide in a few weeks if was going to have any at all. It was time to think and tune to a guide that had more answers than I did.

For ten years I had been trying to get in touch with my Source, my spirituality. I'm sure we all have it. It's kind of a voice that helps us know what to do and what not to do. I had been developing my Source for over 5 years and I was starting to get confident in its advice. I don't mind telling you I was scared, uncomfortable, alone and scared. As I was going through this whole process, something seemed wrong, out of kilter. It didn't make sense and my Guide was pushing me to do some alternative thinking.

As a youngster growing up I had idolized my Uncle Glen Gardiner. He was a doctor. He had a new Cadillac each year and a beautiful wife who was warm and caring. The few times they came to visit our family they always brought batches of candy. We rarely had candy in our house, so when my uncle and his wife (my Aunt Bertha) came to visit, it was a big treat. Going to visit them was an even bigger deal. They lived in one of the big three-story houses near Chicago. There was plenty of great food, warmth and caring. Yep, I was going to become like my Uncle Glen. I was going to become a Doctor.

One fall they came for a visit. My brother had been playing football and managed to split open his head right at the eyebrow. Uncle Glen to the rescue. I watched Glen sew up my brother. Watching the blood ooze out of the wound was bad, but watching the needle pierce the skin was too much for my ten year-old mind. Blood and guts have bothered me ever since. So much for doctoring. But he was still one of my heroes as was the whole medical profession. I give credit to Dr. Williams, our pediatrician, for saving my one year-old daughter's life. The miracle of birth occurred in the sanctity of the operating room, not to be viewed by the expectant father. I still have a great respect for the medical profession and their ability to set bones and fix broken hearts and replace livers. I'm sure you've seen the articles and admire their skill as I do. Cancer, TB, and other long term diseases seem to be another matter. When I was told I had *hemocromatosis*, I asked what part diet and lifestyle had played. "Nothing" was the reply. You have to give blood and come see US for a check-up and your number. It just didn't make sense to me.

When I had put on some extra weight a few years earlier I became concerned about my blood pressure.

"Yes, it's up, start taking these pills. You'll probably need them the rest of your life."

"Diet?"

Oh yeah, reduce your fat intake and exercise might be good.

Take pills the rest of my life? Turn the management of my life over to people in white coats? Be under their direction and control forever? That didn't suit my style. I changed my diet, started running and two weeks later my blood pressure was 120/80 and the germ of mistrust had been planted. I had been abused and I would never trust "them" again. I threw the high blood pressure "medicine" away and realized I was responsible for my health and no one, NO ONE was going to tell me what to do without me questioning their methods and their self interest—greed.

I went back to my motel room and started thinking. What if it's positive? What will I do? How will this change my life? I had a son named Christopher living in the city. I called him and told him there might be a chance of cancer, would he like to know about the outcome of the testing?

"Yes," and would I like to have dinner with him and his girlfriend Kate and her Aunt Lou and Uncle Mike Arrington?

"Yes." Dinner was wonderful. Actually the service was terrible, but we made light of it and had a great time. The conversation turned to health issues, and Lou explained that she had had a real run-in with the medical community. She detailed part of her story. It was fascinating. I explained that I was an author and that if she would like to tell her story someday, I would love to help her. I told them all about the cancer "test" and they all said they were interested in the outcome, and would I keep them informed. I realized this was polite conversation. What I didn't realize was they meant it. "They" would change my life.

Over dinner the Arringtons explained their golden tan. It was from carrots. They explained their lifeglow and healthier outlook. Lou had been to the brink. In coming back, she developed a lifestyle that proved to be a benefit, if not a lifesaver, to her husband

Michael. I listened carefully to their views on disease and cure, on what you take into your body and how it impacts wellness.

Two days later I got the news on my voice mail. The results were positive. Could we set up an appointment to discuss the results and treatment.

Oh God, this is it. My knees were weak so I sat down. I suddenly felt rotten all over. My mouth got dry. My stomach started to turn. I put my head in my hands and started to cry and swear at the same time. I was alone, and there was a giant bear that was attacking me. I had to win or die.

A month or 6 weeks before, I had met a tall lovely blond lady in Houston. Nancy had been a stewardess for Braniff Airlines. She flew for them for five years and after returning to get married she arranged a sweetheart deal that allowed her to travel for free. She took advantage of it. She traveled around much of the world and met bright attractive sophisticated people (mostly men) from Buenos Aires to Stockholm, from Hong Kong to Athens. I had been alone for almost five years and liked it that way. I was working a consulting job in Houston and was staying at a corporate suite on the northwest side. Well Nancy was not just a worldly bon vivant, she was also a healer. The touch of her soft hands made me feel immediately better. I trusted her touch and treasured her companionship. But it was time to go to Denver for my check up.

I sat in the silence of my room, the different emotions rolling over me, self-disgust, anger, fear, disillusionment, sadness...great sadness.

"I really don't need this," I said to myself. "But I've got it, so now what? I need healing."

I asked my guide if it would be a good idea to call Nancy. Yes, do it now. I picked up the phone. She said she would come. The appointment was set with the doctor. The war was on.

The Going

I arranged an appointment with Dr. Alexander Goodblood on the 17th of January, 1996. Nancy, my friend, had come from Houston to Denver to be with me. The appointment was late on that winter's day. It was cold and windy; a 6-inch snow had fallen and more was on the way. My son Chris and his girlfriend Kate had said they would come but were not there at the appointed hour, but they arrived shortly thereafter. The weather had slowed them up. Goodblood sat on his side of the desk in the "daddy" chair and the four of us were across from him in "baby" chairs. His side of the desk was free and open, we were bunched together. He was in control.

He explained that there were measures that described my prostate condition. On an ABCD scale, which described my condition, A was a BB-sized cancer. B was a pea, C was a grape and D was a plum-sized cancer. These are not his terms but this is what it looked like to me. Mine was a B, so my cancer was as big as a pea. The second measure described how contained the cancer was (1-4). One (1) was completely contained, four was it had burst the prostate and was on its way to everywhere. Two and three were in between. I was a one, completely contained. That sounded better than the alternatives. He said my liver and chest were good, and that my "acid phosphates" were normal.

"What are the options?" I asked. "Let's get to it." Cut, burn and poison was the answer. They didn't use those terms but that's what they meant.

Surgery, chemotherapy and radiation were the therapies he was referring to. In chemotherapy, they use a series of chemicals to eradicate the affected area. In radiation therapy, they use rays to burn out the affected area. In good old surgery, they get a very sharp knife and cut out the affected areas. In many cases, they use a combination of the remedies to solve the problem. All the methods are invasive. They invade your (my) body and destroy a part of it. This type of medicine always has a downside where something bad always happens. It's called "consequences" or "side-effects." You have no doubt heard of people losing their hair or throwing up or the biggie—death. John Wayne did death. Millions and millions of people do death. *After* the chemo, after the radiation, after the surgery, they do death. After the time and pain and agony, after the hope, after the thousands or millions of dollars, they do death. Not rest in a mountain meadow with birds singing by a stream, but doped-up, twenty-four hour hospital bed, slow, painful, lonely death. The Goodblood plan was to put me in a hospital, go to surgery, cut open my cute little tummy (I don't know this for sure, they may go up their favorite orifice) and cut out my prostate. *If necessary*, they would then apply some radiation.

Okay, friends, these are your choices. What would you do? You would probably ask him the consequences. He would not start with the bill, but sooner or later you would know about that part. How about the bad stuff like death? Not very likely—less than 50% in the short term. Just kidding. I don't think he mentioned it.

He also explained that there was a 10% chance I would wet my pants which I hadn't done in years and a 50% chance of impotence. Well, I am certainly not the best-endowed man in the county, but when Nancy heard that figure, she started shaking her head. If I had radiation that figure went up to 70%. Her head started moving demonstrably back and forth. Well, I knew where her vote was. Dr. Goodblood was not making any friends in her corner. She gently squeezed my leg letting me know:

A. She cared.
B. She didn't want to find a pee bottle there.
C. She wanted night-time action or our deal was done. Well, if not really C, she did want to explore other alternatives. So did I.

We didn't talk money but it is my understanding the removal and treatment of a prostate can run over $20,000. Since my insurer was State Farm there was a good chance Dr. Goodblood would be paid. Let's see, 10% to 25% for Doc Goodblood—well there I was $2000 to $5000 on the hoof. Guess what his recommendations were.

A. Shop around and get a better price.
B. Consider going to Mexico and see what they can do.
C. Change your lifestyle—diet, exercise, herbs, minerals, read books on alternative medicine which will all cost peanuts.
D. Get started immediately with Saw Palmetto and vigorously seek natural means of healing my prostate.
E. Proceed with a radical prostatectomy.

The wind came up and snow swirled around the window on the office wall and he said 'E.'

"That's what I do," he said. "I do it five days a week." No doubt he was filling the Lutheran Hospital "toxic waste" cans with removed prostates, but one of them was *not* going to be mine. I smiled, reassuring Nancy. I put my hand on her thigh and gave a soft squeeze. We looked into each others' eyes and the search was on for C and D.

Chris and Kate asked enlightening questions designed to find out about the real problems in his recommendations and what were the real improvements that can be made from a healthy lifestyle. The real answer was "cut." If you are a retired general and desert storm hero, or coach of a NFL football team, "cut."

Night had come on and I looked out of the window at the snow-swirling darkness. I saw the reflection of us in the window. This was not a team effort. It was him against us. Chris, Kate, Nancy and me on one side of the desk and him on the other. When the conversation started, he seemed bigger, more important than we were. As the meeting came to a close, *our* team seemed bigger, more powerful, more animated, more determined to find a way, not just follow the way. Dr. Goodblood looked smaller and tired. He had come up against a group that wanted to solve the cancer problem, not just fatten his bank account. He couldn't care less about me. He was a medical practitioner and he was after my prostate. Not once did he initiate the subject of diet or beverages or exercise or stress relief.

Several times he referred to data he apparently was well-versed in, data on the consequences of different combinations of surgery, chemotherapy and radiation. If it had been his prostate—and someday it will be—what would be his choices? What would his wife want him to do? Would he research some alternative medicine for himself or his father or his brother?

Medical doctors are well-educated, if not bright, people. Fifty years ago, they were almost all truly dedicated to curing disease and saving lives. Chicago Hope and E.R. notwithstanding, it appears to me that medicine has become a business. Whether the current practitioners like it or not, it is going to change. To keep their patients, they're going to have to go back to doing what is best for the patient and consider all the alternatives, including alternative homeopathic, naturopathic medicine.

If we don't know what causes cancer, and we don't (or 'they' don't), and the statistics of cutting or not versus death are almost the same, why are we cutting? Money, money, money, money, money, money.

Medical school is expensive. Inventing new medicines is expensive, and you out there with your prostate are going to pay. The American Cancer Society and its related and associated organizations take in money, hundreds of millions of dollars. They have thousands of employees and they want your prostate. The doctor did not drive a 10 year old Chevette to work. He wants your prostate. For years insurance companies said "These are the good guys. Use them, we'll pay for it."

From what I read, some of the insurance companies see a train at the end of the tunnel and now they're looking at alternative, homeopathic, natural medicine too. Why? Because regular medicine is bleeding them to death, and they've got kids in school, too.

It's tough going against the system. At this point I am paying for all of the costs of doing it My Way, while still paying my premium to good old State Farm. I am going to ask them before this project is over, if they would rather spend $2000 and have me get well or $20,000 or more, and have me eventually die. Because that's what happens, friends, if you don't cure the source that caused the cancer in the first place it will come back.

I don't want to put myself in the role of a researcher here, I am NOT. Nor am I a medical authority, but I do read and you do too, right, I mean I think you're reading right now! And all the stuff I read talks about a percentage, and it's a healthy one (excuse the pun) of the treated cases, where the cancer comes back and the patient, after spending beaucoups bucks - dies. I'm going to die, and unless I miss my guess you're going to die too. What you and I are trying to do is:

A. Have a healthier, happier more comfortable life.

B. Die in our sleep or in the sex act, whichever comes first.

C. Help other people with both A & B.

As I mentioned before, I have a coach. Answers from my coach/guide used to take days or weeks. Now the answers come in microseconds. So, not only did Nancy's hand on my thigh help me decide, but my guide said, "Don't let that man touch you again." And I didn't. I want to confirm right now that if I have an acute medical problem, I will seek traditional help. If my leg is broken, I will not expect herbs and medications to solve the problem. But for systemic and chronic problems, I am going for a "natural" solution.

Am I Macho Man or not? No. I'm not. Having grown up in an M.D. family (my uncle was a surgeon) and world, it was with great reserve and even trepidation that I decided to go "natural." The whole system from the medical community to the drug companies (when was the last time you saw an hour of television without an advertisement for some kind of drug?) to the insurance companies (when was the last time you saw an hour of television without an ad for some sort of insurance?) to the finance industry (when was...) is involved with fixing your medical problem and paying for it. It was great that Chris and Kate and Nancy all backed my decision to go natural, but let's face it, if I was wrong, it was me alone who would pay the price. I know that I would be missed, but you know what I mean. Don't you?

I had used my guide for everything from which lane of traffic to get into, which car to buy, should I say what I am thinking, to should I ask Nancy for a dance the first time. Maybe it is a cop-out but I don't do anything of consequence without checking it out with my guide. I'm doing it right now as I write these lines. I can't say it's for everybody but it sure works for me. My life has become less troublesome, more successful and healthier. One quick clue. My guide is not a policeman. His job is not to keep me from experiencing pain and failure, but I do have less of them and fewer dire consequences. Isn't that what we expect from a guide—to learn, but survive?

Kate called Lou. Lou said start with *Saw Palmetto*. I happened to be in Boulder so I went to Hanna Krogers' store. I bought Saw Palmetto, opened the bottle right there and started taking it. The clerk asked me if I had ever heard of Hulga Clark and her book *The Cure for all Cancer*. There are a lot of cures for cancer books out there, and this is one of the more radical. She says that parasites are a causal link in the cancer chain and if you get rid of the parasites, you stop the cancer. Many experts will tell you this is a vastly oversimplified solution, but all of them would agree that parasites are almost surely part of the problem. I asked my guide and he said go for it. I bought the 3 required herbs and started my treatment right then and there. The three herbs are hard on your system but they do kill the parasites. I saw the evidence.

Around January 20, Nancy and I drove back to Houston together. On the way she asked if I would like to stay at her place. Am I living right or what? I tried being coy for 1.4 seconds and then said, "OK. Let's try it." Nancy had some needs that she thought I might help with. Now don't get the wrong idea, I am more than a sex object. I knew her as a true natural healer and she could help me to health which she had in spades (or should I say hearts).

I'm sure many of you have heard of Dr. Gray and his colon cleansing system. That was next on the menu.

Dr. Gray has been recognized as a world-class expert on the colon and its impact on health. Colon cancer has been on a dramatic rise the last several years. We have been filling the colon with 80% high fat, high starch, low bulk, low roughage. This three foot hunk of large intestine has been storing gunk for up to as long as we have been alive. I have seen pictures of what some people have been storing and it is not pretty. Thank goodness pictures don't smell. So Dr. Gray's book gave me the short course on the colon, why we need it, what it does, how we abuse it and what to do about it.

His solution is a solution of corn husk powder and pills containing herbs. The two have a synergistic effect that if used for an extended period—three months—will clean out the colon and eliminate the parasites that hang out there.

I have had several friends recommend colonics. This is a kind of backflush for the colon. I wanted to try a much less mechanical solution to my problem, so I stuck with Dr. Gray. I know it sounds crazy, but many "users" wax poetic over how wonderful, clean and empty it leaves them feeling. My colon has had quite a bit of traffic recently and I will probably leave the wonderful pleasures of the "Big Flush" to phase two, if necessary. At this point, if I can't take it camping, I don't want to do it.

So after three months of Dr. Gray's cure, I was feeling lighter, more energized and healthier. I changed my diet, reduced meat by 90%, eliminated BEER and all alcohol. I reduced fat by over 60%. Salt went down 30%. Sugar is my toughest item, but I reduced it by over 30%.

What we put in our mouths has to be the biggest cause of prostate cancer, the fact that Dr. Goodblood all but ignored it notwithstanding. Just think about it. How does bad stuff get into us? We've got this great skin that keeps bad stuff out. Even our eyes and ears and you know what are protected. So if bad stuff gets in, it's pretty much got to be from what we breathe or put in our mouths. Isn't that why you and I took that last Tums? That bad stuff didn't jump into our stomachs. We put it there. I did, anyway.

I remember reading a book years ago that said we are carnivores like lions and tigers and that therefore we should eat meat, lots of it. More current studies say we are really more like herbivores and that therefore we should eat vegetables and fruit. I have been in the process of changing my "vore" loyalty and identification from meat to veggies and find the change to be healthful, less expensive and less gassy. My friends say "Bravo."

It seems we work our whole adult life to be able to afford to eat (and drink) anything we want. Then,' when we can afford it, our bodies can't handle it. Bummer. Well, I found out that not only were the veggies and fruit better for me, they also tasted great. I found a restaurant in Houston (named Houston's) that had a vegetable platter that tastes wonderful and is cheaper than the meat plates.

I found that as I get off the meat and fried foods, I could taste more of the other foods and they tasted better. My friend Lou Arrington tells me I should eat 31 different foods a day. That seems like a lot but a good salad can have 6 or 8 or even 10 different foods in it. Each different food brings something good to the party.

It's amazing how many delicious foods you can find after you get off the meat, potatoes, lettuce routine. I cruised the aisles at the food store and found dozens of foods I hadn't even considered before. It was easy to reduce fats because there isn't any of the bad kind in fruits and veggies. Salt and sugar went down easy, too. for the same reason. Breads were another matter. I liked rolls and croissants and anything else that is made of flour. The problem is that it makes me look pregnant. That doesn't go with my haircut. There are a half-dozen alternatives, including corn, that work okay, so for awhile at least, I'm giving up bread. The wheat problem is not part of the cancer but it is part of me and that makes the challenge more... more challenging.

When a person wins a car race, they spray champagne all over each other. I consider this to be a really dumb practice, but celebrations with alcohol of one kind or another is a worldwide tradition. Well, I have to wait two years until my PSA gets to 2.5 or less, then maybe. In the meantime, I have been introduced to all kinds of fruit drinks (as I recall, wine and champagne are made of fruit) that taste absolutely delicious and serve the celebration function just fine.

Coffee is a favorite beverage, not the regular stuff at Denny's or McDonald's, but Starbucks. The problem with coffee and regular tea is that they drain my body of minerals and I'm spending $2 a day to put extra minerals in my body. Kind of stupid to defeat my recovery. So I have decided to wait a year for coffee, and then only in moderation. That means one or two cups once or twice a week. In the meantime, it's Earl Grey and his herbal cousins.

The hardest part about diet change is the stuff that just seems to slip in. When I was paying for a relatively healthy lunch recently, I took a free little bag of M&M-looking things. Before I could say "Liposuction," they were down my throat. For one week I compiled a diary of *everything* I ate. It was amazing at week's end to see how much stuff I ate that:

Wasn't on my diet.

Wasn't really enjoyable.

Wasn't worth the carbs or calories or fat or anything else for the enjoyment it brought.

When I ask myself, "Is this really worth the food content and the money?" before I eat something, the answer is frequently "It's okay but *not* really worth it." If it is, I eat and enjoy. My size is slowly coming down. My goal is about 170 on my 6'1½" slender frame.

I started running again 1½ to 2 miles three times a week. I got a mini trampoline and I think that will work better.

Exercise is a key ingredient in conquering cancer because exercise:

Relieves stress built up from life's regular frustrations quadrupled by having the stress of cancer laid on top of it.

Strengths the body and its immune system to conquer the disease.

Creates a positive mind-set that I am *doing something* to beat this killer.

Provides positive feedback for me. I like myself when I exercise. I feel good about me. It's like a pat on the back, which very few of us get with any regularity. Exercise, even moderate exercise, does that for me.

It makes my body look and feel better. It gives me an image to see that's more worth saving from death or deformity. I can't see me at the gym working out and looking good except for that pee bag strapped to my leg. I don't want to put down the guys that go that route or wear diapers, but I'm going for the approach that doesn't include that in the plan. Sorry, Dr. Goodblood.

Sex was tripled to once a month—only kidding, but Nancy and I usually go for a half-hour walk 5 days a week. A lot of cancer patients want to shut people out and go through their process alone. Not the best choice. Actually, all parties benefit by joining the fight. Everyone involved takes a closer look at their own life and lifestyle and usually:

Finds more to appreciate about what life has given them.

Adjusts their consumption habits to insure their health and longevity.

Reaps the benefits that come with helping another human being through a rough spot. It engenders a great feeling of being a good person.

The numbers are compelling, comparing cancer patients who are alone in this quest for survival, and those that have a support family. Those with a family not only do better on the live/die scale, but those that do survive also have a much better and easier time of it and have happier birthday parties and anniversaries later.

I started telling some key people about my problem. So I took the chance at rejection, sticking my neck out. I am more than pleased with the results. Sure, some people that I thought would help or care didn't. But others *did* care and their support added new flowers to my garden of life.

I stuck strictly to my Hulga Clark and Dr. Gray programs. The toilet is not my favorite place for personal viewing but if you doubt you have parasites, take the tour. I lost ten pounds in a month and I'm sure much of it was from what had been eating *on me*.

The stores and libraries have scores of books on cancer. The bibliography at the end of this book lists quite a few. They fall into two general categories. Category One is success stories of people who used the system to solve their problem. Most of these stories depict heroic efforts, much pain, money and survival. As Dr. Dean Adel said on one of his recent radio shows, "...blood cancer was a death sentence. Now there is a fifty percent survival rate." The system has saved millions of lives. What is not said is that millions of the millions later died of the disease they "*survived.*" Reading stories like these is immensely important because it shows man's (and women's and children's) drive to survive through months and years of pain, humiliation and loss. A few will tell the story of how their survival completely wiped out their assets and left them alive but broke. The cost in many cases is "all you've got." In too many cases, when the money ran out, the treatment stopped. The patient died. Eighty per cent (of those who died) died of the same disease they had "survived."

Category Two of books deals with alternative medicine. This category focuses not on solving the symptoms but on determining the cause. Putting on skin grafts is the first system's method of treating sun-damaged skin. The second system's method is to stay the hell out of the sun. If you believe in a divine power, you have to believe that we have built-in solutions to every problem, from mosquito bites to cancer. This category helps you invent the solution to your problem in yourself. Read and find hope...in yourself!

Chris and Kate got engaged and I was invited to the wedding at a beautiful mansion on a mountain near Denver. I asked if his mother (my ex-wife) was going to be there. He said yes. I started getting cold feet. Kate said she would protect me. Chris said he would protect me. Nancy said she would protect me if I would take her along. I went. They all protected me and I came away unscathed, but I will confess I was the first to leave after the wedding dinner.

Mike and Lou Arrington were at the wedding. They were charming and pleasant as could be. They extolled the virtues of Arizona, as a Naturopathic Medicine State, and offered their hospitality should I choose to go there for treatment. They talked about a Dr. Lance Morris,[1] an NMD they recommended highly.

Arizona has become the mecca of those who used to go to Mexico for treatment. Your federal and state governments—dominated by medical, insurance, drug and finance companies—have driven people who were living in the U.S. to Mexico. Some went to Germany for treatment, but Mexico was close and cheap. The problem was that most of the patients who went there were either almost on their death bed or broke or both. Hulga Clark's book details how many were saved and many were not by her clinic in Mexico just south of San Diego. Arizona and a few other states saw the problem and decided to license naturopathic doctors. This meant that the doctors could prescribe medicines and really get about solving the patients' problems.

Depending on who you talk to, the Mexican facilities are either bogus or life-savers. From stories that I have read and people that I have spoken with, they have beautiful facilities that do good work. But bring your wallet. Your insurance company as of 1997 will probably not pay for any of the costs. They will pay huge amounts for using the current system but not for holistic cancer treatments. This is in a state of change. Arizona is helping to lead the way.

For me, things were moving ahead nicely. I met a young fireball named Karen who wanted to be the "producer" of my seminars. This had been very much of a sideline for me, my real living was provided by an incentive awards company that I own. With Karen's gusto, I did a couple of radio shows and made the cover of "Center Point" magazine, extolling my personal excellence and the benefits of my ten minute seminars. At the first event the place was packed. Maybe it had something to do with the fact the seminar was free. We did sell a few copies of my book, *The Velvet Glove—Building Relationships That Fit Like A Glove*. The fact that Mark Victor Hansen's endorsement was on the back probably added to its pull. In the seminar I included a short spot about "how we are guided and protected—how to make a right decisions every time." I was surprised at the positive feedback and

---

1. Lance J. Morris, NMD, 1601 N. Tucson Blvd. #37, Tucson, AZ 85716. (520) 322-8122.

expanded the topic at the next day's seminar. I combined the 10 minute (how to know you have met your ideal partner in 10 minutes) seminar with the "How to make right decisions" and concluded the two with "How to better know how to love." It went great. I felt great. My cancer was drying up. The parasites were leaping out of me, and it was getting time to find out how I was doing.

In late summer, America West was doing $100 round trip flights to Tucson. I called Lou. She and Mike graciously offered their condo, their car and their golf cart if we would come to Green Valley, 30 miles south of Tucson. We took advantage of their offer.

In mid-August, I called Dr. Lance Morris, N.M.D. FANCM, Naturopathic Physician and Diplomate in Family Medicine, for an appointment. I saw him on September 9, 1996. Nancy went with me. Dr. Morris' office nestles inside a complex of homeopathic healers of one sort or another, just north of downtown Tucson. The receptionist handed me the regular paperwork bundle to fill out. About fifteen minutes later, this smallish bundle of energy introduced himself as Dr. Morris. We spent quite awhile talking about me, my medical background, my lifestyle, eating and drinking habits, emotional stresses, and even my spiritual life and values. Nancy and I both liked him.

The whole approach was "we" (he and I) have a problem here and together we will solve it. It would be a team effort. I asked him about his background and why he chose natural rather than standard medicine. He thought it made more sense to cure the cause rather than symptoms. His schooling as long and arduous as an MD's but with a different emphasis. He was looking to find the cause of the cancer and then solve that, rather than repairing or eliminating the wound (in this case, my prostate).

He took blood samples and we made an appointment for a live blood examination. He and I would both look at my blood together. He would show me what was good and what was not. We set up a time for the next day.

Lou and Mike Arrington not only gave us the use of their lovely condo in Green Valley, looking out on the beautiful mountains that surround the community, but they also gave me their beautiful new Jeep Wagoneer to drive. We took advantage of their warm generosity and took a short tour around the local area. It is easy to see why the area is booming. It is a golfer's paradise, a deluxe development that they live in.

Lou invited us over to her home a mile or so from the condo where we were staying. The Arrington home was magnificent, with emphasis on the natural. Modern adobe might describe the design but it was light and warm and friendly, loaded with plants inside and out. Lou had her own victory garden, Victory for victory over poor health and disease. Her large variety of plants grow year-round in the fabulous climate of Green Valley.

Since Lou had a life and death battle with not only T.B. but also the medical profession, she embarked on a lifestyle that returned her to health. That lifestyle keeps her and Mike in the healthiest of conditions. They both look ten to fifteen years younger than their age. They both possess more energy than almost anybody else. Lou has dedicated her life to learning about health and healthy living. She has started her own book about her battle with T.B. and how she almost lost. Eventually, with good luck, guts and determination, she won.

We toured some of the local area, discovering how the vegetation changed with the topography. Cacti filled the deserts while trees of all sorts covered the mountains. Flowers of different sorts mixed in between for color and visual flavoring. Is there a plan here? It sure seems so. If there is a plan here for balance and beauty in the universe, perhaps there is a plan for balance and beauty in the universe of our bodies. It just makes sense to me.

The next day we went to see Dr. Morris at 9 o'clock. The staff took a sample of my blood, put it on a slide and placed the slide under a special high-powered microscope with two sets of lenses. Dr. Morris and I could both see the blood sample at the same time. He sat on one side of the instrument and I sat on the other. Focusing on the blood sample called a *live blood analysis*, he explained to me what it all meant. The microscope had a pointer in it that the viewers could move around. He pointed out details of my blood that he said were good and some that were not, that needed changing. After ten or fifteen minutes with me, he gave Nancy a tour of my blood. I got back on the microscope for Phase Two. He scraped one piece of the blood sample glass against the other to make the sample thinner. We could now see more detail, how the red and white cells interacted. We could see the platelets and the comparative numbers of white and red cells. A third thinning showed us even more of the activity.

We then sat down while he showed us pictures of healthy blood and cancerous blood. Fear welled up in my chest, but I had to ask him, "Do you see my cancer?"

"No," he said. "If there were any cancer there, we would see it in the blood. In fact, with this test, we can see evidence of cancer up to *ten years* before it would show up with regular testing."

"Ten Years?" I repeated. "Why isn't everyone using this stuff?"

"Naturopaths do," he replied. "This is what we do, and then we see the problems and treat them."

My God, I thought. What would happen if all the clinics did this? What would happen if all American men could know in advance that they were getting cancer, that what they were doing to themselves was causing cancer? Wouldn't it be great? What would they and their families and their employers do to change things to stop the onset of this disease and save millions of lives and billions of dollars? What would you do, Mr. American man? How about your wife, your family, friends and employer?

Well, if lifestyle (deathstyle) is causing cancer in the first place, why don't we change it now for everybody?

Let me explain again that I am not a medical practitioner or a researcher. I am a business consultant and problem solver. There seem to be two distinct and different methods of getting at the problem of cancer. Allopathy creates a kind of war zone (me against me) kind of thing. I will identify this problem as a disease and I will fight it (suppress it) until it finally wins and I die. Like my blood pressure problem, I will take these pills and fight the problem for as long as I live. In prostate cancer, I should cut out, irradiate or chemo out the disease and keep the symptom (enlarged malignant prostate) suppressed until I die.

Allopathy vs. Naturopathy

ALLOPATHY	NATUROPATHY
Germ Theory	
Single Etiology	Multi-faceted Etiologies
Symptoms = Disease	
Physicians as Pathologists	
Law of Opposites	Law of Similars
SUPPRESSION	CURE

Naturopathy asks, "What is the cause of the symptom?" and then finds it, changes it, recreates balance and says "Go on with life." In the case of my blood pressure problem, I didn't need a pill and the services of a physician. I needed the services of Me. I needed the services of Will Power. *I* changed my diet and eventually lost fifteen pounds. I started an exercise program and two weeks later tossed out the remainder of my blood pressure pills because my problem was gone! I have never had a blood pressure problem. I had a *me* problem. Can you imagine the time and money I would have spent taking medication and treatment the rest of my life for a non-existent blood pressure problem?

I am coming to conclude that *Medical Insurance* is the biggest disease we have in this country. "*If* Insurance is paying for it, I'll just go ahead and take the treatment." Is this crazy or what? *We* are paying for the premiums, whether by check or payroll deductions or unpaid job benefits. "If I don't have to pay for it, I'm going to go ahead and have it done." How many times have you heard this? You are paying for it either in direct charges or by taxes. When will we start taking responsibility for our own lives, especially heath care and its costs? When will we start taking responsibility for our health? The catharsis that changed my life was cancer. Goodblood and Company were the messengers but it was me—I was the one—who caused the disease and no amount of medical care paid by my insurance or not was going to cure me. Goodblood wanted me to be his financial slave. I, through my insurance or whatever, would be paying him to *suppress* my cancer as long as I lived. Morris wanted to help me find what was causing cancer in the first place and *cure* it.

When my catharsis hit, happened, struck, I was floored, frightened and frustrated. Because I was a road warrior, any system I developed to change my lifestyle would be thwarted by a lack of geographic balance in my life. I was at the other end of the spectrum from Mike and Lou Arrington and their beautiful stable environment. Nancy not only came to the rescue with a beautiful place to live, she also brought a farm girl background of healthy lifestyle habits. She ate moderate amounts of basically healthy foods. Her whole lifestyle was one of hard work, saving and healthy moderation in most things. Exercise was not her strong point.

Mike and Lou are the epitome of what to do and how to do it. They bought food almost exclusively from a store that sells almost exclusively organic foods. They both exercise over three days a week. When they travel, they take organic food and produce and proper water with them. Lou constantly researches new recipes. Every meal I had there represented a textbook example of how to eat healthy. She served fresh foods from her garden right out the door almost every day. They built a proper water system. They subscribed to magazines and other sources of information for healthy living; their mailbox overflowed daily with it.

Just in the short time I was there, she put out lady bugs to keep bad insects out of her garden. No need for pesticides. She received special worms to treat the soil so it would raise better crops. No need for chemical fertilizer. They join organizations that do healthy things. I was invited to a vegetarian pot-luck dinner, a delicious opportunity to exchange recipes and ideas.

So with this "Model Health Home" as an example, I decided to move step by step to being as close as I could come to the Arringtons in *my* lifestyle. Nancy concurred and we started becoming regulars at the Whole Foods Cocktail Hour. The Whole Foods Grocery chain with seventy stores nationally sports a fruit juice bar. At one store in Houston, they have a cocktail hour where fruit and vegetable drinks are 75¢ off. Most of the material I read extolled the virtue of juicing. Juice Man became a cult hero of the health set and the sale of juices and juicers has grown explosively. Nancy and I started having rendezvous at the cocktail hour at Whole Foods, swilling down twelve ounces of carrot juice or some other healthy concoction.

My biggest hurdle was sweet rolls and nut breads. Unfortunately, right across the aisle from the fruit bar reposed the bakery section with the most delicious assortment of rolls and breads you can imagine—free samples on the counter. This was Nancy's weakness, too. We had a choice: to be the source of each other's strength or each other's weakness. Strength won and we reduced our consumption fifty percent. I guess life's greatest challenge is to work hard enough to afford most of everything you want and then have the willpower to have it in moderate amounts.

I note here a product and person who very likely delayed the onset of my cancer and may be a force in the future for cancer prevention. Three years ago, I met a Dr. Walter Connard, a chiropractor from Lincoln, Nebraska. Dr. Connard had developed a formula consisting of aspartated minerals. He asked me to help market the product. I started taking it myself. My energy increased dramatically. My PSA numbers dropped. It was one nightmare after another getting the stuff made. Dr. Connard tired of funding the money-losing operation. He finally lost patience with the whole business and shut it down. He is currently exploring new solutions to the manufacturing question. So far, I'm not satisfied, but if and when they get going, I will forward the information to the holistic health community and in particular to Dr. Morris.

My final meeting with Dr. Morris ended on an upbeat note. The results of my tests would be finished in a couple of weeks. We arranged for a phone interview.

Did I survive cancer? I don't buy that philosophy. I am pro-active. If anything, I conquered cancer. But I don't consider this a victory. It is only a step on my path. Did Hulga Clark and the parasite killers kill cancer like she said it would? I don't know. Did Dr. Gray help? Probably. Did the lifestyle change help? Yes, but I have to get a lot better. I have to eat organic foods and drink good water and exercise and meditate and do fifty-one percent. Dr. Morris makes a point that we can't eliminate all the problems all the time, but if we can eliminate most of the problems—diet, emotions, exercise, environment, structure, genetics, and pathology most of the time (fifty-one percent)—we can have a pretty good chance at successful healthy living.

I asked Dr. Morris, "Do you think I ever had cancer?"

He said, "Probably."

So here I go. Am I clean? No. I have some other physical problems that I need to solve and resolve. I should probably get a house one of these days. Nah. I've got my great car and there's always the Big Blue 6. Tom Bodet left the light on for me. There's even some talk that you might want to hear more about this "health" stuff and how it is part of making perfect decisions and finding the right mate, and hiring the right person.

Nancy and I took the Red Eye back to Houston. It was tiring but I'll tell you Houston looks different when you don't have cancer. I walked taller and felt calmer. This huge weight was off my shoulders. As the sun came up, we drove home to Nancy's from the airport. I started feeling grateful. Grateful to all of the people along my cancer path who reached out to help. The word love went fleetingly across my consciousness. Maybe that's it. Maybe I love these people.

A couple of weeks later on September 23rd, 1996, I had a phone meeting with Dr. Morris. He confirmed that I did have some problems with my adrenal gland that would take some work, most importantly, no or greatly reduced wheat flour.

I was *given* (we know that means pay) a series of medicines to help improve my blood and make me like a ten year-old. You will never guess how this medicine is ingested in my system. What is with me and the medical community? okay, I had thirty suppositories to take over ten weeks. My rear end was apparently the thoroughfare of choice for my medical problems. Other bloodwork numbers for cancer looked good and my hemocromatosis was determined not to be family-related, so my boot-destroying brother was mistaken.

As a side note, apparently using my boot leather to make his first slingshot was a lifecourse-setting event. After ROTC at Wisconsin, my brother went into the Army and became a unit commander of an atomic cannon, one of the largest slingshots the world has ever seen. Way to go, Bob.

Well, it sure looked like I had won and without the invasive procedures Dr. Goodblood had wanted. I wonder how State Farm will treat the business. I'll let you know before I'm finished with the book. How I will stay on top has a lot to do with how I manage my stresses—physical, mental and emotional—which impact my life. A lot of that management has to do with:

1. Knowing the personality profile of the person I'm dealing with.
2. Using an internal guidance system to help make decisions.

I'm supposed to be an expert on #1 and I'm getting very experienced in #2. Let's check it out.

Well, folks, as a new member of the I.C.C. (I Conquered Cancer) club, I'll have a few ideas for you on staying the course in the next chapter. See ya.

Stress That Kills

Okay, I've spent a lifetime getting cancer, six months or so getting rid of it, and now I have to keep it gone—walk the walk.

Dr. Morris lists seven factors that influence our "getting" a disease. I have rearranged their sequence to make a point:

1. Genetics
2. Pathogens
3. Environment
4. Structure
5. Diet
6. Exercise
7. Emotions

1. There is very little at this point in my life that I can do to change my genetics. They are what they are. I feel good about the "hand" I have been dealt, but it doesn't make any difference. I've got what I've got, whatever it is, and I've got to make the best of it. *I'm not in control of my genes.*

2. Pathogens are in the air, water and ground that are a part of my world. As long as I live on the planet today I'm going to be exposed to pathogens. *I'm not very much in control of pathogens.*

3. *I have some control over my environment.* I can sit in the non-smoking section, live in the less polluted part of the country/city and, to some degree, influence how my environment impacts me.

4. I have five separate and interacting lives: my Business life, Financial life, Personal, Health and Spiritual lives. *I have a pretty fair amount of control over how I structure my five lives,* what I prioritize and how I live them. The world of traffic jams and weather still impacts my day but I'm still fairly in charge.

5. *Diet is pretty much in my control,* not completely, but certainly more than my genes. Foods today are pretty clearly labeled and I know what stores sell what and what restaurants sell what.

There is a limited choice, but food is portable so I can take my choices with me.

6. *Exercise is something I can almost completely control.* If I want to and have the will power there is almost never a day that I can't get ten minutes of some kind of healthful exercise. There are any number of devices that I can use where I am, and there are many others that I can take with me, especially my legs. If nothing else I can walk, or in a bad neighborhood, run. Sometimes exercise can be done sitting still. So if I'm not getting my reps (repetitions), it's strictly a matter of will power, and to a tiny degree scheduling (structure).

7. Emotions are the toughest of all. *I have much control.* But in my case, and frankly in most people, it is the greatest cause of illness and probably accidents also.

"He's worrying himself sick."

"He's going to worry himself to death."

"I'm worried sick."

You know the routine. I've got total control over my thoughts, yet I worry about all the stuff from the first six factors over which I have less control. There is no way that I will ever have a day in which one, or more, of my five lives (Business, Financial, Personal, Health, Spiritual) is to some degree out of my comfort zone. That's life. At least it's my life, today.

There are many good books available on how to handle stress. I would like to deal at some length about two problems that cause difficulties (stress) for me and probably for you.

The first is "Who is this person and how can I deal with them in a way which will assure both of us the best possible result?"

The second is "I have dozens, scores, hundreds or even thousands of decisions to make, choices to determine everyday. How can I do a better job of making fast, accurate, fair decisions that I won't later regret?"

Difficulties—stresses—within these two areas set off chemical reactions in our bodies that, when caused persistently and consistently, beat up our immune system. And that, friends, makes us susceptible to cancer. So here is how to *reduce* the problem.

"Who is this guy—how do I deal with him?"

A statistics professor developed what is called the PEPOLE Profiling System. That is not a mis-spelling, rather it is an acronym for a system that clearly, quickly and simply defines our personality profiles. This is not a simple set of pigeon holes that we fit into, rather a very sophisticated method of defining who we are. Even in its simplest form it has over one thousand different profiles and in its broadest measurements shows *over* ten million different profiles. My effort here is not to make you experts in the PEPOLE System, but rather help you become familiar enough with it that you can determine who you are dealing with and therefore be able to deal with them more effectively. It's not very complicated to use. It's very accurate and to you, my valued readers, it's free.

The first person we want to deal with is you. The basic premise is that whatever is, is perfect. Like flowers in a field or our thumbprint, all of us are a perfect us. There is no preferred or best profile. We are all made different and we are all made perfect. Repeat: we are perfect.

We have different instruments that we use to get to our quantification of the amount, or intensity, of the six traits that we measure. We are going to use the simplest one here. The six traits we are going to measure are: Power, Extroversion, Pace, Organization, Logic and Energy. We are going to measure them in the simplest of terms. (See Table below.) Are you on the left side of the trait, in the middle, or on the right side? Remember, there is no right or wrong, no better or worse, no more or less good. Whatever is, IS.

So start with yourself. Circle *one* word on each of the six lines. On the Power line, are you mostly cooperative? If so, circle the word "cooperative." If you are mostly dominant, circle that word. If you are *neither* mostly dominant nor mostly cooperative, then you are in the middle, so circle the word "middle." The form looks like this:

PEPOLE Survey

Are you:

P	Power	COOPERATIVE	Middle	DOMINANT
E	Extroversion	RESERVED	Middle	OUTGOING
P	Pace	FAST	Middle	PATIENT
O	Organization	CREATIVE	Middle	STRUCTURED
L	Logic	FEELING	Middle	FACT
E	Energy	LITTLE LESS	Same	LOT MORE

Here is what a profile might look like that has been filled out:

PEPOLE Survey

Are you:

P	Power	COOPERATIVE	Middle	DOMINANT
E	Extroversion	RESERVED	Middle	OUTGOING
P	Pace	FAST	Middle	PATIENT
O	Organization	CREATIVE	Middle	STRUCTURED
L	Logic	FEELING	Middle	FACT
E	Energy	LITTLE LESS	Same	LOT MORE

In this case the respondent thought he was more *cooperative* than either dominant or in the middle. He felt mostly in the *middle* on Extroversion. In Pace he felt he was neither fast nor patient but in the middle. On Organization he was not creative nor in the middle but rather he was *structured*. In Logic he was mostly *feeling* oriented and his Energy was a *lot more* than most people.

Of the first four traits (Power, Extroversion, Pace and Organization) the one that is to the right is the most important. If more than one is to the right then a selection must be made. *Which* of the two or three is most intense? That *one* is the most important trait. The trait *of the first four* that is to the left is usually second-most important, depending upon how important Logic and

Energy are. There can be cases where the first five traits are all pretty close to the middle and Energy (the sixth trait) is very much more and therefore that can be the second or even the most important trait that describes a person. "He's kind of a middle of the road guy but he has energy that just won't stop."

So, if the reason for learning this stuff is to reduce stress, then how do I use it? It's simple: give the person what they want. Let's use the profile example above. The trait farthest right of the first four was Organization. This person wants needs and likes "structure." Give it to him. He likes all the details in a question before he gives an answer. Give him all the details. Be specific. Be exact. If this person is being asked to buy a stove or a car give them all the details about the stove or the car. If this person is being asked to prepare dinner for guests, he wants to know how many people, what do they like to eat, when is it, where will it be held, what people are wearing, what are their backgrounds, where should the food be bought? No loose ends. This is not the person you tell to "just put something together, it will work out okay." It may work out okay but it will stress this person out of their comfort zone, maybe a lot.

The second most important trait here (because it's farthest left of *the first four traits*) is Power. This person is cooperative. They want their world to cooperate. They like teamwork and security. These are *not* risk-takers. What others want to do they will want and want to cooperate with.

Physical size, mental make-up, and other trait placement has nothing to do (no correlation) with personality traits. A cooperative person can be big or little, bright or dull, structured or creative, patient or fast-paced or any other combination of physical, mental or personality profiles. The thing he isn't is dominant. He doesn't want to take charge or be the boss. He is not a sales closer. He is not an "in your face" kind of person. And regardless of his physical size or mental abilities, he will be stressed-out and fail if asked to do these things.

So, it's that simple. The person wants what is circled and is frustrated (stressed) if he doesn't get it or is asked to be the opposite. The opposite of cooperative is dominant. The opposite of structured is creative. Are we together?

Let's try mine and then I'll give you some real life examples of how people succeed and fail because of their profiles. Here is my profile shown in the Table below.:

AUTHOR'S PEPOLE Survey

P	Power	COOPERATIVE	Middle	DOMINANT —▶
E	Extroversion	RESERVED	Middle	OUTGOING
P	Pace	FAST ◀—	Middle	PATIENT
O	Organization	CREATIVE	Middle	STRUCTURED
L	Logic	FEELING	Middle	FACT
E	Energy	LITTLE LESS	Same	LOT MORE

There's a problem here. There are two traits to the right and two to the left. The arrows show which is the most intense. So yours truly is a dominant (farthest right) fast-paced (farthest left) person. Both Power and Extroversion are to the right. I asked the person being profiled (in this case me), are you more outgoing or dominant? Dominant I said, so an arrow was drawn to the outside (away from the middle) to show that I was more dominant than outgoing. So now we know the farthest right trait. Are you more fast-paced or more creative, I asked myself. I'm more fast-paced, I politely responded, so the arrow was drawn away from the middle to the left. So my farthest left trait is Pace. This is a dominant, fast-paced person. "Do it my way—right now." The farthest right and the farthest left together represent about seventy percent or more of who a person is. So by using this simple little card you can be very close to understanding who the person is, and therefore what please (motivates) him and what frustrates (stresses) him. And this friends is a major cause of "what ails you".

But why am I doing this stuff? This is nuts! Am I supposed to run around with a little card or a piece of paper and say "Hey, before I let you know who I am or allow you to do business with me or be my kid, I want to do your profile?" But we are already doing something like this. It's called conversation. And we're learning a whole lot of stuff, but we don't know who we're talking to. Is this dumb?

After thirty years of marriage, you do not know who you are married to. You don't know your parents, friends, associates, boss, kids, anybody. I have done many, many thousands of these profiles and I have asked thousands who had some meaningful person in their life was (wife, for example). I asked just in the most general terms who the person is. Are they dominant, cooperative or in the middle? Are they outgoing, reserved or in the middle? Are they fast-paced, patient or in the middle. It is *very* important to give three choices (right, left or middle) for the system to work. If you ask "Are you structured or creative" the system breaks down. If you ask "Are you structured, creative or in the middle" it works like a charm.

Out of many thousands, can you guess how many correctly guessed the other, six out of six traits? Zero. Nada. Niente. None.

So that's why you should do it. So you know who you are talking to and supposedly understanding. And that will reduce stress. And that will help you keep your little walnut-sized prostate. That's why!

But there's an easier way to do it. Use a napkin. That's why this was originally called the "napkin test." Here are some ways of getting started:

Example 1. "Say, Bill, I saw this test that's supposed to help me understand you better. You wanta see it?"

Example 2. "Honey, I was reading about this survey that is supposed to help me listen to you better. Let me show it to you."

Example 3. "Johnny, I found this survey that is supposed to help me understand my children better. I'm going to ask you six easy questions about you."

Example 4. "Jim, I read about a survey that I found helps me understand people's communications better, and know where they're coming from. I'll show you how it works."

Example 5. "Honey you are a gorgeous lady, and I want to do the best I can at getting to know you. I just read this fabulous book by this handsome, brilliant world-famous author, Eric Gardiner, and he says we can be happily ever after if I do this napkin test thing with you. How about it?"

I know you will develop your own opening strategy, but these have worked for some people.

Example 6. I say something like "I use the PEPOLE Profile to get to know people. In terms of power are you dominant, cooperative, or in the middle?" After you do it five or ten times it becomes almost automatic. What's more you become antsy until you do it because you *know* you *don't know* who you are talking to.

Is it worth a try? I hope so. If you can remember the word PEPOLE—like a dog peeing on an electric pole that really shocks him—then you can whip out a napkin or any convenient piece of paper and write down one side:

P
E
P
O
L
E

Then write in the words:

P Power
E Extroversion
P Pace
O Organization
L Logic
E Energy

Then lay out the grid and fill in the choices.

P	Power	COOPERATIVE	Middle	DOMINANT
E	Extroversion	RESERVED	Middle	OUTGOING
P	Pace	FAST	Middle	PATIENT
O	Organization	CREATIVE	Middle	STRUCTURED
L	Logic	FEELING	Middle	FACT
E	Energy	LITTLE LESS	Same	LOT MORE

If you can't remember all of this, copy the layout in this book. If you want a little business card-sized version for yourself and others you care about to use, get in touch with us. We'll sell you some, cheap. I really want you to have this. It will change your life for the better.

I have done this profiling thousands of times on napkins and scraps of paper. It shows whomever I am doing it for that I care about them. I care about them and me. I know that without this I am wrong about who they are and therefore I am wrong about me. I don't want to be wrong about me, period, especially when it's so easy to be right about the whole personal interaction.

Here are some examples of the impact that knowing a person's profile had on relationships. We start with the premise that almost everyone thinks that almost everyone else, at least in our own culture, uses their common language the same. Stop means stop. Go means go. Black means black. I love you means... Hold on! Not only are there different interpretations of words, we all speak a different language. All 260 million Americans (as of 1995) speak a different language, and the personality profile has a great deal to do with what we mean when we say something, or for that matter, the way we behave.

Two brothers-in-law were trying for years to get along. To say their relationship was strained puts it mildly. Brother-in-law 'A' thought brother-in-law 'B' really didn't like him very much. 'A' felt he was treated brusquely and was not liked. When he discovered that 'B' was a fast-paced, very reserved dominant person he realized that 'B' treated everyone that way. 'A' was an outgoing extrovert and thought everyone was nice to everyone unless they were mad at them. 'B' wasn't being bad or nasty to 'A'. He wasn't mad at 'A'. He was just being himself, but in 'A's language the words 'B' used meant he was mad. He wasn't. When 'A' understood this he became understanding of 'B' and their relationship became closer, more harmonious, and less stressful.

Two people met at a big social event and dance. They were both attractive and attracted to each other. Good-looking, smart people with similar background and values. He wanted something to happen. She wanted something to happen. It didn't happen. They had an okay evening and made a date for lunch the next day, but by that time they were terribly aggravated with each other.

"Would you come on?"

"Would you slow down?"

He was a very fast-paced person who wanted a fast-paced companion. She was a very patient person who wanted everything to go slow and easy. Fortunately, they were so bad for each other it ended before it ever started. Before marriage. Before kids. Before divorce.

We certainly wouldn't try to match a team of horses that didn't have the right temperament for each other. Same thing with sled dogs. Why do we try to couple ourselves with people we don't match with? Because we don't know how not to!

Jim tried to have a family with Lucille. He was a dominant, dominating person. He dominated her for ten years. She was a dominant person who hated being dominated. She grew to hate him. Divorce fixed everything. They're both broke and hate everybody. Why didn't they figure it out beforehand? Why didn't someone tell them it wouldn't work? No one knew how.

Bill and Andrea were married for eighteen years. Life was good: house, kids, cars, boat. Then they were getting divorced. Why?

"I can't stand it anymore. I love him but I can't stand him not making up his mind about anything."

"I can't stand her. I ask her if she wants to go to a movie and she asks me what I want to do. She won't decide on anything."

Bill and Andrea were both cooperatives. They both wanted someone like Jim or Lucille to decide on things, to take charge. A counselor using the PEPOLE Profile System showed them the problem. They both decided to be a little dominant, taking turns making decisions that affected them both. They moved to a giant castle in the clouds and...No, but they did stay together and continued on with their life together.

Do problems like this cause stress, enough to cause problems to the immune system and increase the chance of *cancer? Yes!*

Marcia had been hiring telemarketers for her operation for five years. Their contract with AT&T depended on providing the services they were *contracted* to provide. It took about 120 people to do the job. They had to hire ten to fifteen people a month just to stay even. Hiring was more than a headache. It was a sword of Damocles hanging over their heads. No hiring = no performance = no contract = no job. This was not "I'd like to"; it was "I have to." They were probably spending over $500,000 a year hiring and training. This does not include the extra amount of deodorant necessary to mask the stress-induced odor for the management team. Stress = Cancer. Are we getting somewhere here?

Yes, we found the problem.

Yes, we solved the problem.

Yes, the turnover was reduced—dramatically.

Yes, we were paid.

Yes, they used less deodorant.

Did using personality profiling (The PEPOLE System) help make the difference? It was *the* thing that made the difference. Marcia was spending a ton of money on advertising, screening, selection and training. She left out *the* most important piece of the job/person relationship: the fit between the profile of the job (at the micro level) and the employee.

If this is so simple, why doesn't everyone and every company do it? Please sit down for the answer.

Just as the people in charge of finding a cheap, fast, effective cure for cancer have a vested interest in *not* finding it, so people who are responsible for finding a cheap, fast, effective method of hiring have a vested interest in *not* finding or using it. If an employee of the American Cancer Society found the answer to cancer in a fortune cookie, what do you think would happen to him and his cookie if he talked? If an employee of General Motors found the cure for hiring and turnover woes in his fortune cookie (which would cost over 10,000 Human Resource Department jobs at GM alone) he would soon be found stuffed inside the muffler of a new Corvette. That is, if he shared his fortune cookie fortune.

Let's face it, surely 50% of the stress of our modern life is generated by the people who have a vested interest in keeping it that way and exacerbating it. How about the I.R.S.? How about... nah, let's not do that here.

Janet (who had a year-old daughter by a previous marriage) went to a dating club to relieve those cold lonely nights. She was, as my Mother used to say, "cute as a bug's ear." After paying $1500 she was fixed up with Alex, who had paid $2500. They had a great date, fell in love and were married. Janet's ex-husband still hated her. He sued them both for custody of his daughter. Neither side won but Alex spent his life's savings, over $50,000, trying to keep his new wife's four year-old all to themselves. What's buried in our past can cause real problems today and tomorrow. Maybe if Janet had used this little PEPOLE survey with her first husband she:

1. *Would have gotten along with him better and stayed married.*
2. *Would have realized that they were never going to make it and never have gotten married.*
3. *Would have done 1 or 2 above and have saved Alex and her exhusband a lot of money.*

As this was some years ago, I'm guessing that both Janet's ex and Alex are well on their way to seeing Dr. Goodblood.

For more information about the PEPOLE system, consult the appendix or read *The Velvet Glove* (see the last page).

One last point (it sounds so simple it seems almost not worth mentioning, yet it is the basic reason we "fall out" of relationships, business or personal). We forget to ask "How am I doing?" I read recently about a woman who was arrested for putting a contract out on her husband. She paid a man to kill her husband. The deal somehow didn't go through and she tried *again*. The man she paid the money to happened to be a government agent and she was arrested. When told, the husband was flabbergasted. He thought, as a couple, they were doing fine! Talk about a lack of communication.

How many times do you see in business places customer comment cards "How are *we* doing?" How are you doing? How am I doing? I know of a woman who was living with a man for over a year. She frequently asked him to tell her how she was doing. Was he pleased with the way things were going? Did he like her? Did he think he was getting his needs satisfied? Yes, yes, yes, yes, were the replies. He was happy. A year later she walked out. He never asked her if she was happy, was she okay, what could he do to make her life and situation better.

It doesn't do any good to have all the tools in the world to solve people problems if you don't use them. The computerized PEPOLE Survey has a stress analysis built into it. (Yes, I did it on one, and yes, I was in the "Red Zone"– the year my PSA numbers shot up and I was diagnosed positive.) If you have concerns about yourself or someone else, it could be helpful to find out:

1. How much stress you have.
2. Where it is coming from.

The PEPOLE Survey shows you. Its also great for high school kids. I had a friend whose son was in the "Red Zone." I told her she had better get help for this kid and fast. "No, Jimmy is just fine." I said "No, he is not fine. He has serious stress and you need to do something about it." She didn't. Six months later "Jimmy" killed himself.

Is it worth saying "Be Nice?" This is not just good for your personal and certainly your business life, but every part of everything you do. When I got my wake-up call with the message "Yes, Mr. Gardiner, your biopsy was positive," life became finite. I realized I was going to die. I beat prostate cancer but sooner or later you and I and "all God's children" are going to die. I decided that I was simply going to spend more of my days and years being nice. I'm not where I want to be yet, but I'm working at it, every hour of every day. It's a lot easier when I go inside and ask my guide, which brings us to the next part.

6 Staying The Course

Dr. Morris made it clear. This was not a game which when won would allow my old lifestyle, whatever that was. Some things would have to change for now. Some things would change forever. What a body was able to withstand or process in 1900 was vastly different than in 1950, even more so in 1995. We used to have soil. It contained minerals that crops absorbed, and then which we absorbed. A funny thing happened from roughly 1850 to 1960: the top of America's bread basket blew away, to be washed down the river, figuratively and literally. Louisiana and the Mississippi Delta grew hundreds of square miles larger, thanks to the transfer. You are the poorer nutritionally for it.

The wind doth blow and the rain doth fall. You have seen films of the dust bowl. It means to you and me that food grown in this soil doesn't have the same nutritional value as before. Without massive amounts of fertilizer, (600,000,000 *tons* each year, it doesn't even grow much at all). No problem. Just keep pouring on the chemicals. One problem. The chemicals are killing us. A tape called "Dead Doctors Don't Lie" making the rounds for multi-level marketing of supplements clearly and effectively states this case.

Organic farming to the rescue. This isn't the only solution but it certainly is part of the solution. Buy organic foods. Go to restaurants that serve organic foods. When possible, use substitutes for foods that you know are bad for you in quantities you eat now. There are substitutes for almost everything from porterhouse steak to french fries, diet cola and pressure-cooked chicken. Many of these substitutes taste delicious. At first, you may find organic foods to be higher priced. If you factor in even a small part of the stomach remedies and other cures that you don't have to buy, and perhaps even a small part of the doctor bills you don't have to pay, you will find organic foods to be a real bargain.

I have not had to take an antacid since I changed my lifestyle. I had a whole diddybag full of medicines. Now I carry vitamins and minerals. I'm not there yet (we never really get *there*) but it is working for me. What you put in your body and don't put in will have a huge impact on how you live and survive.

Is this good business for the purveyors of a healthy life style? *Whole Foods, Inc.* of San Antonio, Texas, now has over 70 stores in ten states. Their stock more than doubled in the last few years alone. *Moveable Feast* is another operation that sells wholesome, organically-grown foods and the lifestyle that goes with it. Throughout the country, stores and shops like these open up to the new marketplace.

More and more resources come online every day. Health magazines line shelves by the dozens. Prices of supplements plummet. Although many suppliers still try to get away with huge markups, buyers shop more aggressively. Even Rexall, one of the great names in American naturopathic products, is on board with Wal-Mart and I am sure many other outlets with a line of economically priced supplements. Look for prices of healthy living to come down as demand goes up. Be a careful and vigilant shopper, though. I recently went to a health fair where a mini-trampoline was offered for a show special of $300. At Wal-Mart afterwards, I found a similar one for $24.95, not on sale.

Organic farming represents good business. The costs of growing are less because there are no chemicals or fertilizers, yet with the proper methods the yields are high. Crop prices at the farm exceed ordinary, non-organic pricing by 10 to 20%. The farmers must feel some emotional dividend for feeding consumers healthier food.

If you are not already buying organic foods, look under the Yellow Pages listings for "Foods—Organic." You will meet new people and start a healthier way of living.

What can't I have? I'm not here to tell you what you can or can't have, should or should not have. I'm just suggesting. I could be totally wrong and pushing up daisies in a few years, but I don't think so. I feel better, stronger and healthier than I have in a long time. What can't I have? I *can* have anything I want, but I now choose not to have coffee, alcohol, sugar or tea, short term so I can have them later. "All things in moderation," said Adam before he ate the apple. Still, it is a line of advice to be heeded, possibly the best advice of all.

You don't have to be very old to have thought about drinking water. In the 50's and 60's, only a small section in the grocery stores was traversed by devotees of different lifestyles who talked about water. Now whole aisles stock water for the masses, in "We've got the world" supermarkets.

What's going on here? Disease, chemicals, toxins, metals, germs, bacteria, filth and death. We've ruined it, folks. You, me, Republicans, Democrats, Independents, ecologists and everyone else. We've put toxic chemicals on our *grass*. We've dumped garbage in our dumps.

We patronize a throw-away society where we buy a ½ pound product in a one-pound package. Remember when you walked out of that fast food restaurant with arms full of packages of food, enough to feed only four people? Well, you're drinking it. Hundreds of millions of tons of chemicals are put in and on the food products we eat each year. Some of it washes off and flows to the sea, along with parts of the Dakotas and Kansas. Atlantic and Gulf seafood ingest it and then you buy them at your local food market only one hundred feet from the aisle where they sell you the water with the stuff filtered out!

We have a problem. I am doing something about it. In the meantime, you have to drink something and most people don't drink enough water. No wonder. Distilled water has no bad stuff but no good stuff, either. We need water—8 glasses a day—and not as a mixer. Most people don't drink that much because it is inconvenient to have to urinate that much. I decided on filtered water. Some decide on distilled.

We should drink less of many things. You know them: coffee (I knew a man who drank 35 cups a day), pop, phoney fruit drinks with less than 10% fruit juice and so on. Don't give up. There are two alternatives.

Number One is moderation. An acquaintance drank a gallon of Diet Pepsi a day. That is a habit. It went with her smoking. Ask if you really enjoy that 3rd, 4th, 5th or 10th cup of whatever, or is it a habit? It can be changed. You don't have to stop. Just get better.

Number Two is alternatives. Great, delicious alternatives don't cause cancer.

Next on the list is breathing. When is the last time you breathed? Probably just recently. New construction techniques and heat-saving methods make our homes and offices more airtight, frequently more polluted than the air of the city we live in.

Twenty-five years ago I had an electronic filter in the house I owned near Chicago. Each month I cleaned it I was constantly amazed how much dirt it removed. Are things better now? Air filters, fiberglass filters, non-allergenic filters and all kinds of others can fit home ventilation systems. I do not want to live in any home without air filtration. Even homes with baseboard heat can have good filtration. Portable units can travel with you. Many of the new cars have built-in micron filters. Ask the dealer.

Heat 10° F Midwestern air to 70° and it becomes dry. It is bad for your entire respiratory system. Humidify it. Treat the water in your humidifier so that you don't spread water-borne diseases, but humidify. I had a chronic sore throat in the winter for years. I went to the doctor for antibiotics. Then I rented a farm house for two years. It had an old steam heat system and I had no visits to the doctor.

Conclusion: If you have air in your home, filter and humidify it.

When you change your lifestyle, you will lose some friends. You will have to make some more. If you decide to stop smoking, you will lose your smoking friends. Your children will still be your children, but your smoker friends will drift away. If you are coupled, it is easier and more fun to change together. Support each other, especially when one gets weak. Many marriages have been strengthened by two people who chose to make positive changes together.

Consciousness is what you think and feel. If you think constructive and positive thoughts, feel good about yourself, you're on your way. I give myself a five to ten minute mind game: "I am good. I am doing the right thing." My higher power wants me to do this thing *to* me *for* me. I can better help others if I can help myself. We get well in our minds first. The whole Naturopathic philosophy rests on the body healing itself. That healing starts upstairs in the gray matter. See yourself being healthy and you will get there. Don't see your self healthy and you will find yourself swimming upstream against the current.

I need to remember that healing is what the body (and mind and spirit) does all by itself. I don't have to tell my body to heal or show it how. It does it automatically. We are healthy naturally. We are doing a lot of things to harm ourselves, but just stopping the bad stuff is a big help to our bodies. I burnt my finger recently, fairly badly. I put on aloe and some other medicines, but my finger healed itself. My treatment helped and I trust speeded up the cure, but my finger with the rest of me did the real healing job.

We are naturally healthy. We are naturally happy and we are naturally successful at doing what we tell ourselves to do. That's just the way we were designed and created. So much of modern medicine is invasive and tries to force a cure instead of letting us heal ourselves. Watch a baby develop. He is naturally happy and healthy and automatically learns to crawl and walk and then run, laughing and happy much of the time. Then, somehow, we get him, and ourselves, off track.

Lastly, I need to refer to my "big guy," my "guide," my "higher power." It took me ten years to get comfortable and confident with the relationship, but now it is here and I use it many times a day. I believe now that we all have a discreet singular one-on-one frequency with a power that guides us perfectly and protects us. I have mine and I believe that you have yours. He, She, It will give you all the answers you *ask*. It used to take me days or weeks to get answers. Now they come in less than a second. I use my guide for every question of every sort in all of my lives—business, health, social, and so forth. In the years that I have been asking, I believe that I have never been misguided. Now, I don't decide anything without my guide. No question or matter is too small. This cancer thing has been no small matter, so my guide is all the way with me.

Here's how I use the System. I consider life one long continuum of questions and choices. Every hour of everyday I make dozens, maybe hundreds, of choices.

> Which desert should I order?
> Which car should I buy?
> Should I try to call or see this person today?
> Is a customer okay or do they need to be contacted?
> Should I ask for the order now?
> How should I price this item?
> Have I made enough entries on this material I am writing now? (Yes.)
> Should I go on to further explain this system now or should I wait? (Now, do it now.)
> How many more pages will I need to describe this process? (Two or three, but more will be needed to describe the career and spiritual uses of it.)

I use the System constantly. Many times it is a kind of question and answer thing and others, the best way to do something, or the answer to an unasked question just pops into my head. I don't want to suggest for a minute that the degree to which I use this is something you should do or aspire to, but wouldn't it be nice to have correct or best answers to many of your life's questions or problems? Wouldn't it be wonderful if we could teach our children the use of this system so they could make "right" decisions when growing up? Don't you wish you had an interior guide helping you when you were a kid? How would your life have been better if you had:

> Made decisions to invest properly in homework time?
> Not made that resentful comment to your teacher, parent, sister, date?
> Not told that lie?
> Not stolen that book, idea, property?
> Taken chemistry or algebra instead of study hall?

If this sounds insane forgive me, but I have been doing this hard and steady for over five years, and the results have been remarkable. Again here are the steps I use:

I pose the question in a clear, positive way.
I listen for a clear, positive answer.
I act with all my ability to achieve the goal, or with full confidence in the rightness of the decision.
I say thank you.
I use the confidence of a positive experience to question/ engage my faith in the success of the next question/ answer.

I know this is not unique to me, it is not even unusual. We have all had enlightening guidance that worked in our behalf. What I'm talking about here is cancer. What is the right road for you or someone you know who has cancer? I now talk to people about cancer almost everyday and almost everyone I talk to knows someone, or knows someone who knows someone, who has prostate cancer. On tonight's news Arnold Palmer was reported to have prostate cancer. As the male population ages every man is going to have a pee bag and there will be millions and millions of horny old ladies because all these old dudes are going to be impotent. Is something crazy here?

So you try using this stuff and you get positive, uplifting guidance that encouraged you to be nice to people, and honest, and whatever else you're supposed to be doing anyway and the world turns out to be a better place. What are we coming to?

I can hear it now, regarding questions on unfair advantage: How can I bet on the stock market, or the football pool, or the Kentucky Derby. I don't think so. How about these?

Should I stop here for gas or should I wait?
Should I give this person a gift or not?
Should I go to New York next week or wait?
Should I hire the guy or not? The PEPOLE System says he's okay, but something is bugging me. Follow your guide.
Should I loan this person the money.

I have known one other person in the last two years who uses his guide as I do. He couldn't live or be in business without it. He uses his guide constantly.

If we all have this gift, why don't we all use it, all of the time? Simple: we turn control of our lives over to other people and institutions. Local, State, and Federal governments spend half of our income. Organized religion tells us what's right and wrong. (Kill those people, they are wrong, evil, or misguided.) Television tells us what to buy and almost everything about everything and everybody. I have not personally met Clinton or Dole. How can I possibly judge which one to vote for? The School System tells us what to do. Our spouses tell us what to do. Our kids tell us what to do (but not mine). Our boss tells us what to do. What is there left to decide? Everything.

> Should I go talk to Michelle's teacher about this, or am I wasting my time?
> Should I say something to this lady, or should I just let her go on talking and then leave?
> This business man has an interesting idea. Should I listen to him or am I wasting my time?
> Is that movie worth going to or is it a waste?
> Do I have to get that muffler fixed today or can I wait till next week?

The help is endless. I have been doing this for years, and it works. Will you at least try it? It will take some of the uncertainty and stress out of your life. It sure has mine.

Remember that "Butter's bad, use margarine" advice? The 'authorities', 'experts', 'US Government studies' and number of other *authorities* have told us something was wrong. Then they changed their mind, or "new studies show...." Now butter is okay, or more okay, or something different from what we the uneducated and uninformed masses know. Are you getting tired of being whipsawed? Are you ready to turn into your own guidance system? It isn't always easy, faith never is, but I did it. I suggest you give it a try. True answers wait.

So it is a whole range of lifestyle items that need to change, from what you eat and drink to what you think and do. *If what you are now doing got you to where you don't want to be, maybe it's time for a new plan.*

Hulga Clark makes two important points in her book, *Cure for All Cancer*: stop using poisonous ingredients and metals.

Stop using all products made with ingredients including the word "prop"—like propyl alcohol. These ingredients poison your immune system.

If you went through your house and garage you would find there are literally scores, if not hundreds, of products that you use everyday, month, or year that are bad for you. They are made of poisons. Do you really think you can spray a room full of bugkiller and breathe it yourself and it not have some effect on you? You don't need to. There are substitutes for almost everything. I got into it heavy right away. I found substitutes for over 80% of the "bad" things I was using. It's really not that big a deal. There are resources in every city with a million people and mail-order houses that ship everywhere. I believe in five years or less the major food chains will start holistic sections in some of their stores. Kroger is already handling organic foods in some stores. Holistic everything can't be far behind. Its simply good business. In the meantime use the resources in the back of the book. The degree to which you need to jump into this depends on where you are with cancer. People I talk to who have no hint of cancer are seeing the handwriting on the wall and are making small but continuing changes. People who are at risk—men over fifty—are getting it and solving the problem before it becomes a house fire.

It really doesn't take a lot more work, just a little research and careful shopping. You won't feel the physical effects immediately, but in time your body will be better.

Smoking isn't worth mentioning. It is a death wish.

For some insane reason tobacco use is resurgent in this country. What I read about it and what I see is this cigar smoking growth is incredible. I personally think it has less to do with tobacco and more a statement about individualism and independence, and not buckling under to the Government. At what cost? The psychological impact is stunning. Smokers are not only consciously ruining their health, but those around them, especially their "loved ones." I smoked a little as a teenager. It was no trouble to stop. From what I read, those who want to, stop. Over 25% of the singles ads in newspapers say that smokers are not acceptable to the ad writer. Is there really any reason to go on?

As I mentioned earlier, Hulga Clark also warns us to get the metals out of our lives.

Most deodorants include aluminum. It goes right onto your skin, into your blood, then into your liver. There are metals in the air, water, food, soil and many of them are bad for you and yes, we need iron in our food, but a lot of metals we get are not the right kind and not the right way. Aluminum cooking utensils and containers give us metal in our food. We're asking our bodies to handle it and they can't. Pyrex and stainless do a good job. Cast iron does not. The point is, these metals put a load on us—particularly the liver and when that gets overloaded it goes to our other organs. Then the immune system breaks down and then the weak link. In men, that weak link is frequently the prostate.

Effective and inexpensive substitutes exist for both the *prop*-ingredients and the metal products. If you have cancer already, it is probably worth getting the mercury out of your mouth.

It costs a lot of money to get all of your fillings taken out and replaced by non-toxic material, probably $300 per tooth. Let's see, ten teeth are $3000, twenty are $6000. What are funerals running for these days? Maybe it would be a good buy. It isn't just dying that bugs me, it's all the stuff beforehand, including that four letter word, pain. I have had my share of it in the last ten years and I want to stay healthy until I die.

Because our food values have been depleted by erosion of the topsoil, we have to take food supplements. I take one called Starlight. I checked with Dr. Morris and he said it was good. It's a multi-level deal so it's probably more expensive than it needs to be. I take the "Lifeguard" and the "Taurus" which keeps me healthy like a bull. It has made things better than before this whole cancer event.

There are hundreds and hundreds of supplements out there and you need to decide on something. Regular food, even "real food for real people" doesn't make it anymore. I think it is important to decide on a regime and stick to it.

Lou takes dozens of pills each day. Some are a form of medication, some are just diet fulfillment. I'm still taking some medication, but shortly I intend to be down to supplements only. Dr. Morris has recommended I stay on aloe vera liquid which I buy at Wal-Mart, for a lot less than some specialty shops.

This is a fast changing business and what's good today can be replaced by new medical knowledge and technology tomorrow. I want to keep my life as simple as possible, so I want to take as few of whatever as I can, and still stay healthy. I have a lot of learning to do. It will never end. But I don't want to be a victim of fads. I will stay with what I am doing until I get a strong reason to do otherwise. In every case I will check with my Naturopath whose job it is to be an expert, before I add or delete anything.

Gentlemen (and listening ladies), I'm just trying to keep it simple for guys like me to live a more complete, healthy life.

Eat right.
Drink right.
Think right.
Exercise some.
Stay informed.

I'll close it up in the next chapter.

From The Mountaintop

Eighty percent of those who *survive* cancer die from it.[1] Wait a minute. I thought that if you survived something, you *survived*. They died from what they survived by surviving the symptoms, not the cause.

Chemotherapy, radiation and surgery do not cure cancer. They burn out, ray out or cut out the symptom. Cutting off your running nose does not cure the cold. Slowly but surely, homeopathic treatments are making their way back into medicine. At a recent health convention in Houston, ten percent of the booths exhibited homeopathic subjects.

As I talked to people about my project, I heard the same questions asked:

"What happened?"

"How did you get rid of it?"

I got rid of it the same way that I cured my burned finger. I did some things that helped and allowed it to cure itself. Our bodies are like that and I believe our lives are like that. If we will listen, the answers are there to cure everything that ails us—physical, mental, emotional, financial, spiritual.

I believe that we are led to the solution of our problem.

I was lead to the solution to my prostate cancer problem.

I took a look at two alternatives and chose what I believe is the one best for me. Most people choose the standard M. D. solution. I chose the naturopathic course.

To review, here is what I did:

I meditated and got direction.

I talked to other resources: they advised strongly to start *saw palmetto*.

I started reading several books at once on my problem.

I confirmed my fears through a physical exam and biopsy.

---

1. *A Cancer Battle Plan: Six Strategies for Beating Cancer From a Recovered "Hopeless Case.* Frähm Anne E. and David J. Frähm. Colorado Springs, CO: Piñon. 1992. p.40

I quantified my fears through the professional evaluation.

I learned through an appointment with the urologist his suggested course of action—surgery, probably radiation, too, and the side effects.

I consulted my team for their input.

I meditated. My guide said no to the invasive procedures, to go instead with naturopathic.

I sought advice from Hulga Clark on parasite cleansing.

I bought Clark's book. I bought herbs and started program.

I read many books, all of which mandated diet and lifestyle changes.

> A. Stop all alcohol.
> B. Avoid second-hand smoke.
> C. Use coffee substitutes in short term (one year).
> D. Reduce sugar; reduce body weight by 10 to 15%.
> E. Begin exercise program (permanent—forever).
> F. Take vitamin & mineral supplements.
> G. Choose organic when possible.
> H. Use filtered or purified water.
> I. Reduce fat intake.
> J. Reduce animal foods by 90%!
> K. Eat healthy:
>   • Grains—40%.
>   • Vegetables—30%.
>   • Fruit—15%.
>   • Fish—10%.
>   • Sweets—5%.
> L. Combine food types.
> M. Drink at least ½ gallon of water a day.
> N. Chew foods 20 times per bite.

Do Dr. Grey's colon cleansing.

Meditate twice a day—"Peace, healing, help my brother."

Find a medical practitioner and determine status of disease.

Reduce bad chemicals by 80-85%.

Get metals out of my life—over 67%.

Be strong in my faith in my "guide."

Reduce stress in my life by:

    A. Using PEPOLE system in all cases. See Appendix for
       how to use the system.
    B. Turn over problems and decision-making to guide.
    C. Make commitment to being less confrontational
       (especially when driving) and more accommodating
       (friendly) to all I deal with.
    D. Where possible, rid my life of stress-inducing thoughts
       and PEOPLE. If it doesn't make me happy, drop it!

Find a higher purpose in life and give 10% of my time to it.

"Thy will be done." The solution to my disease/predicament/ difficulty is in "His" guidance. It is really hard, especially for a *dominant* like me, to give up control. "I did it my way" embodies the creed of the American man: we conquered the West and landed on the moon and got prostate cancer. I wanted the disease to be eliminated my way, on my schedule and with me getting the credit. It doesn't work that way, folks. This whole exercise in healing requires giving up control and letting *"...thy will be done."* Nothing I can do will speed up the process. I can help nature repair the damage that I have done. I can give back to my body the things it needs and stop doing things that damage me, but I don't do, and surely the doctors don't do, and drugs and medicines don't do the healing. It was deigned (created) that way by a higher power. My task at the time and for as long as I live is to tune in to that higher power in a concentrated focus at least two times a day. My job is to give over my will to his guidance and let him show me the way. I saw a show recently where the speaker talked about life choices being fear or love. I don't know as much about love as you do, but I do know about fear. I know that when I am not in touch with my guide, life is like walking on a high wire. I feel as if I can fall off any minute. I am worried about the sharks in my life and retribution for my past mistakes. When I tune in, I feel grounded and guided. I still have the symptoms—a pain here, an ache there. "Oh, my God. It's coming back." Then I go along inside and say, "Thy will be done." I go along in my day and do the best I can, doing what I'm guided to do. A big part of that guidance is this book. I have spent well under $1,000 on medical help and prescriptions on my treatment. My first and most important goal, my guided course, is to help some of you see an alternative to the invasive course of surgery. This writing that I do is part of my treatment. It is what I do to fulfill "Thy will be done."

Is that it? Is that all I have to do? New things come up every day. Choices are made every day. I have a weak link and it is ready to jump up and knock me down or kill me every minute of every day. In Air Force boot camp, they told me what to do, what to eat, drink and think twenty-four hours a day. I had very little personal freedom. When we got a half-day off, the enlisted men would go over to the snack bar and pay for what was free at the chow hall and drink two day's pay of 3.2 beer. Now it has come full circle and I am my own First Sergeant. I have to be in charge of me. I have to make all the decisions, with one major change. If I got out of line in the Air Force, I could go to jail. If I get out of line now, I get confined to a much smaller cell, a pine box.

So I don't look at this disease as a sentence. I look at it as a loud wake-up call to get in line and live life as I am supposed to. Life's road has narrowed from the road it was two years ago, or twenty years ago, or forty. Somehow the *straight and narrow* has some real benefits. I can live healthy, alert and unencumbered by excess. I don't need antacid pills or cold remedies anymore. I don't need morning after help. I won't get the jitters from too much coffee or sugar or wine or flour or anything else. The Universe is already delivering people to me who feel the same way, so I can see a house filled with healthy, less baggage-filled friendships, probably some very special ones.

People like you and me read books such as this to find help for themselves or someone they care about. Start with yourself, whether you have cancer or not. Start with the little PEPOLE survey and confirm what perfect profile you have been blessed with. Look in the mirror and see that perfect body. Maybe it has a few extra pounds or wrinkles but you earned every one of them. Whether 6 or 60, you have had a whole lifetime of experience that no one has had. You've already written your own book. Maybe it isn't published yet, but you've experienced it and you've learned from it. The concept of forced retirement at 65 or 70 ranks among the dumbest waste of resources imaginable.

And think of all the good stuff you've got inside. Sure, we've all abused our bodies but you've got a great body on the inside, too. With a little work, you could look like you want within two years. Not two months. Yes, two years. With any of the diet regimens out there, you could be going anywhere you want, doing anything you want to do in two years. I belong to a ski group that travels to a different place in North America each year. We don't ski very well but we sure have fun. When it is my turn to cook, I will cook vegetarian and they will love it.

If you are an American man, you don't have a choice. You are going back to basic training and learn to live right or else it's peebag time. Foregoing that, the boys in the band say you're going to die (and not a happy death, either). This is apparently the weak link now. It's amazing how fast the species adapts. In two or three generations, we may be sporting new and improved prostates that can take the bad stuff, get along without the good stuff and handle the stress. In the meantime, "it's you and me, babe" and we've a choice: mend our ways or become fertilizer.

If someone had told me twenty or thirty or forty years ago what I was doing to myself would lead to cancer, I would have changed. If they had told me just to modify and reduce the abuse I was doing to myself, I probably would have moderated. And if they had told me that I would have to be operated on (etc.), I certainly would have modified my intake of fats, booze and lack of both veggies and exercise. I am not the smartest guy around but with those choices, I would have chosen a more modest approach to living.

That's the main message here. If you don't have a problem now, modify your life and live a long, healthy existence.

I found that the healthier foods are really quite delicious. Going to healthier foods will not sacrifice enjoyment. If you live like most people with a stove, oven and refrigerator, you will find all the ingredients readily available in most cities. The Yellow Pages list health food stores, good referral sources for organic foods. If you are careful, two of you can eat as cheaply as one, or less than you are spending now. Beans and rice are among the safest staples of this lifestyle. How expensive can this be? Crazy as it sounds, some truly delicious renditions for rice and beans abound.

Exercise is not an option, either. Do it or die!

Someone invented the wheel and since then, we have been doing everything we can, to do nothing. We are almost there. The owner's manual for a Model T must have been very slim. Some new car owner's manuals reach 100 pages or more, some even heading for 200. All this to not do anything. Even eating properly, you will have to exercise or blob out. The tough part is to do something. Maybe that is what is good about cancer. We get so scared that we do something. We start living a life that we are supposed to just to survive. Instead, we couch out. We get so sick of everything that we spend the last few years of our lives in hospitals or nursing homes. 'Go, Baby—get cancer,' the best recovery program going. *If* you live, you will *really* live! Dr. Morris talks about doing fifty-one percent. He would prefer us to do one hundred percent, but if we just change most of the seven things (diet, emotions, exercise, environment, structure, genetics, pathogens) most of the way, we have a chance. The more, the better. But let's face it. You and I love butter cookies. Life has to include spoiling ourselves just a little.

It is not easy 'being green.' It is still hard to get the right foods, especially at restaurants. Far less than 1% have organic foods. Water is easy to get but air is still unhealthy. Supplements are easy to get, but hard to get people to act nice to you. It is even harder to get me to act nice to them, especially if they did something like cut me off in traffic or crowd in front in line at a checkout counter. It is hard to turn off the television which shows dumb programs biased against men. It is difficult to drink eight glasses of water a day and to excuse myself to go pee. It is really hard to give up some of the stuff I really like to eat and drink, but so far I have lost twenty pounds. I can run faster. Exercise is getting to be okay and life has a whole new set of priorities. I sleep better (melatonin). Sex is better.

It isn't how much I eat. It is how much I want. It isn't how much I earn. It's how much time I want for my friends and myself. It isn't how much I want to buy. It is "How little do I want to cart around?" It isn't about my gold ring. It is about how I can help you get yours.

Lastly, it is about all of us getting along.

Our government isn't going to help. They're still paying people to grow tobacco and taking fifty percent of our income to do it.

Religion isn't going to help. Please don't be offended, but I don't trust any religion to help. Today's paper reported a Moslem fighter killed 14 women because they would not put veils on their faces. Islam is the fastest-growing religion.

Families aren't going to help. They can be a great resource for some people for some problems, yet they too may let you down.

Who, then? You, then! You have a candle and you have a match. When you light your candle, I will see it and ask, "How can I help?" Other lost and hurting souls will walk out of their darkness and say:

1. I hurt.
2. How can I help?

Then you and I will hold them and help them and love them. You know how it goes. People get a new energy based on helping others. You will meet them at the health food store. You will meet them at vegetarian dinners. You will meet them at concerts, at a tire store or at a workout center. Cancer could be the greatest thing that ever happened to you. It could be the source of a whole new lifestyle and a reason to be. Is this the dumbest thing ever? From tragedy, great good can happen.

I hope to God I made the right choice about my treatment because I'm going with it. I'm in charge. Nobody's stickin' no more probes up my you-know-what and nobody's cuttin' my nuts off.

Thank you for buying this book. Thank you for joining me on this journey. I would love to hear from you whether you think I'm right or wrong. My light is on. I want to be your friend, just like Barney.® I don't care what color you are or where you are from or any of that stuff. Come on in out of the dark or cold and be my friend. My arms are open.

Uh-Oh.

WHAT WOULD I HAVE DONE IF?

This is not a make-a-choice-and-stick-with-it kind of situation. I did not give Dr. Goodblood the finger and tell him that I never wanted to see him again. I politely suggested that I was going to think it over and decide. If my number had not been satisfactory or encouraging, I would have gone shopping. Hundreds of urologists an be found in the telephone book. I would have found one more suitable. Some books suggest building a team of health practitioners who would help me.

One thing I would have done for sure is just what I did: I would (and did) change my lifestyle. I dropped dead tomorrow of whatever cause, the advice in this book can be life-saving for some and certainly life-enhancing for most, if not all.

I will check myself on a continuing basis to monitor how my decision is faring. Are my PSA numbers continuing to go down? Is my Live Blood Analysis continuing to show improvement? Is my body shape good or getting better? Am I feeling good about me and what I'm doing? What is my guide saying about my course?

I'm still scared. I will be until my PSA is under 3 and my weight drops to 180 pounds. I'll still be scared until I learn enough to trust my higher power and stop being scared. My head is my biggest problem. I want to be free of concern, but maybe it's the good old fear that keeps me close to the fire and doing a really good job of what I'm supposed to do. Maybe fear is nature's way of keeping me in line, a gradual process where I feel a little better and then a little less afraid. I'm smart enough to know I have to behave or I'll be back in the pot again.

So, behave better
A little less fear
better feeling
Continuing good behavior

> better feeling
> less fear
> good behavior
> better feeling
> less fear

Sooner or later, the symptoms go away and so too the fear. How long this cycle lasts, I don't know. I'm guessing about two years. I'll let you know.

If I had a friend or brother who had a problem like mine (and who hadn't cut up my boots), I would say study. Consult your inner voice but study the options. A powerful medical community exists out there and it wants your prostate. In many cases, they don't want to tell you the full possibility of the downside. I am not a professional medical practitioner. You need to talk to more than one professional. If I were buying a house or a car, I would certainly look at more than one option. This situation is certainly more important than either buying a house or a car. So get ready to do a little shopping. This book portrays some of alternative medicine and its many choices. At this point, I don't even need to say please. I'm sure that you have read enough to know that there *are* choices. Seek out a naturopath, at least on the phone! I believe that in another ten or fifteen years, the debate about a naturopath or not will be a moot point. All doctors and hospitals will have at least some function as a naturopathic healing service. In the meantime, "It's you and me, babe." At least consider the alternative.

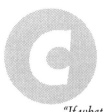

Conclusion

"If what you are now doing got you to where you don't want to be, maybe it's time to change the plan."

Like the five fingers of my hand, there are five elements to my conquering cancer.

Stop the bad stuff. Food: change the diet, reduce fat and dairy products and white flour. Use organic foods when possible. Beverages: eliminate alcohol, caffeine and soft drinks. Metals: change cookware utensils, anti-perspirants and metal dental work. Chemicals: get rid of household cleaning products and replace with natural substitutes.

Start the good stuff. Food: use whole grain cereals and breads, fresh fruits and vegetables (organic when possible). Beverages: drink treated water for drinking and rinsing foods. Drink real fruit and vegetable drinks, not just the 10% or less varieties. Supplements: take daily supplements of vitamins and minerals.

Meditate. Ten minutes twice a day. Program yourself to live a happy, productive day. Program your sleep to be restful, healthful and peaceful.

Exercise. Park at the edge of the lot and walk to the door. Walk up stairs (don't use the elevator). Join a hiking, health, exercise or athletic organization. Breathe deeply, laugh and have fun.

Be a tree. Trees give shade, provide meeting areas and sanctuaries to animals, and protection from the wind. Have you seen a lone tree in a field with animals standing in the shade? Do something nice and out of the ordinary every day. Smile. Hold the door, pull over a lane, let a person in front of you—just to be nice. You will like yourself better. Be a tree.

A word came to me in a dream last night. The word was "Help!" I asked my guide if there were some significance to the letter and here is what I got:

H   Health
E   Energy
L   Love
P   Peace

Isn't that what we're all looking for? Don't we all want or need help in our own lives? What good is living if we don't have the good health to enjoy it? We need energy to translate our health into doing something that will benefit ourselves and mankind. Love is the glue that holds it all together. Sooner or later, we had better be doing it for love or the value of what we do crumbles into dust.

I recently talked to a lady who was losing a business deal. She called a friendly competitor to get the deal and give her a piece of it. Do we all need our own piece of the deal or can we just give it to someone and wish them love and peace? When was the last time you had a really good night's sleep? When was the last time you took time for yourself by yourself for a peaceful stroll in the woods or garden? What is the point of all our own stuff if we don't have peace?

So I wish you all peace and love and energy and health. I am very grateful that I was able to h e l p.

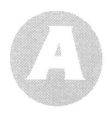

Afterword

by Chris Gardiner

It did not seem important to me at the time, but it is fascinating how life and nature seem to conspire together. A coincidence of weather and circumstances forced me to go slowly in all ways, while driving, while dealing with business, and with the final stop of the day, our appointment with the surgeon.

At 10° in Denver, the world is very quiet, except for the sound of a person moving through it. On my way through the world that day, my father had called to tell me he had come across a block in the road—he had cancer.

With the exception of the sound of my boots across the snow, the world had given me a time of silence to consider his situation. I have taken the time in my life to find many places of contemplation (the last guy down the hill at the end of the day, alone at the top after 8 hours of climbing to 14,000 feet, and other lonely pursuits) but the walk from the car to the door of the doctor's office was a very silent, somber experience.

My best case scenario always allows me time to prepare for an upcoming life event, this time, there was no time. I did not have the confidence that would normally be at my disposal and felt completely unprepared. I had a general understanding of the issues placed before my father, but very little understanding of his feelings toward his crisis. My brief addition to this work is focused on the single concept that helping anyone close to you through a personal (even life-threatening) problem is not as difficult you think.

In my new best case scenario, it is really pretty easy to be a part of critical success in the life of someone as long as time is taken; to understand what the hell they want when all is said and done. I had it easy in some senses, because my Dad is quite forthcoming when it comes down to it. The basic keys to my assistance came from listening to what my Dad really wanted to do, and to educating myself on what was realistically possible. There may be less than a great correlation between my dad and the rest of the people on the planet, but in describing him briefly, my small part in helping him get through a tough time might be of some use to someone faced with wanting to help, but not sure what to do.

The Thrillseeker Syndrome

My college schooling in Finance illustrated the concept of a risk-adjusted rate of return where higher risk is rewarded theoretically with greater reward relative to low risk endeavors. This idea also applies to pursuit of life issues where taking a chance (i.e. starting your own company, leaving the corporate world behind, flying kites during electric storms, etc.) has resulted in some of the great success stories of history.

My dad has applied them to the art of vacationing. I can't recall a trip that had even the slightest intention of being planned, other than generally what continent we would be going to and whether to bring swimsuits or skis. This was, we were told, to increase the opportunity for adventure and without question, our family has endured and delighted in some epic travel experiences. Some folks go to Disneyland, planning for weeks in advance on the magic of meeting Mickey; we would get out of school at 3:00, be in our airplane by 5:00 and proceed to "go west... somewhere... we'll know when we get there."

I have had some of the most daring, exciting times of anyone I know in the company of my father, experiences that are difficult to appreciate unless you have lived them. My father and I have been speeding wildly down remote mountain roads (and crashing), flying a variety of amazing aircraft to wherever we felt the urge (and crashing), racing formula cars on twisting, demanding race courses (and crashing), blazing our way down tortuous ski slopes (and... well, you get the picture).

I have always been fond of my dad's thirst to live life fully, and have, with the caveat of trying to be less in harm's way, continued the family tradition toward adventure. I have even come to understand to some degree my father's seemingly incomprehensible need to pass cars on onramps to the freeway, to attempt to set lateral g-force records in rent-a-cars, and his need to weave his way through rush hour traffic to receive the coveted first-to-the-tollbooth trophy. Although it has cost him some weighty traffic tickets (and one might guess an ex-wife or two who grew distant via the white-knuckle highway), it is his essence, his chosen way, to wildly travel the road through the world and he would be less true to himself to be otherwise. This is not to say that my dad is foolhardy or reckless, he is really just less risk-aversive than most people.

It was in light of this personality trait that my dilemma arose when considering what to advise to him after the diagnosis of his cancer. This was not a case of a bent fender or a sprained ankle. As I walked through the frozen stillness to the health expert who would dictate the only way to keep my dad on the planet, it came into my mind that my old man was a "go out in a blaze of glory" kind of guy and it seemed unlikely he would opt for treatment that would prolong his life if it meant living with infirmity or dependence.

Based on what I knew about prostate cancer, the only options for cure did indeed include a good chance of random loss of body functions. The risk of the cancer spreading would be weighed against the possibility that the patient would lose a life of freedom and independence. In my father's case, I was guessing he would be inclined to take his chances fighting the cancer instead of submitting to surgical procedures. It was with these thoughts in mind that I walked into the office. It was soon thereafter that I learned where the real battle exits in the world of cancer cures.

The Salesmen

Almost everyone in my family makes their living in the sales arena and it is a pursuit that we all understand and appreciate. I am very familiar with the basic concepts involved; prospecting, qualifying, presentation, overcoming objections and closing, to put it briefly. The subtlety of a good salesman is an effective tool to use as it encourages the buyer to pay less attention to objections and move toward accepting the deal.

I have not personally read the Hippocratic oath in its entirety, but I can't recall any specific instruction to the physician concerning marketing or anything to do with increasing market share. As it has unfortunately become the case with many of the classic social charters from the past, this oath simply could not have anticipated what the present world has become. The reality of what the physician faces today became very apparent after talking to the urologist/surgeon my father had chosen. The up-to-date doctor is well prepared to sell what he supplies. It was naive of me to think this, but my expectation was that this man, regardless of how his revenues would be effected, would be the last person to engage in selling tactics. I expected an unbiased appraisal of what the possible treatments were and their rates of success and risks involved.

In all fairness to the physician involved, he did provide a perfunctory list of other options and a variety of tables listing rates of success. As the conversation unfolded, however, I noted a pattern of conversation that felt remarkably familiar. Each mention of the alternatives to surgery were skillfully avoided as far as detail (sales rule: don't focus on your competition). His explanation of his cure process was well prepared and presented in an almost infomercial style (sales rule: a high quality presentation sells). The relative likely outcomes related to loss of bodily functions as a result of having surgery were skillfully downplayed and expertly deflected (sales rule: overcome objections). He emphasized the available schedules for surgery in a creative and friendly way, offering to set the appointment up while we spoke (sales rule: close the sale!).

The whole appointment was well executed with one major exception, the seller wasn't listening to the buyer. This physician was selling his ace card, certainty. His purpose was to pound away at the concept that surgery was the only certain cure. The consequences of this procedure were for the most part ignored, but for the buyer in this case, they were more than just side effects. It seems irresponsible to me that the focus of this conversation was to sell only surgery. In the commercial business area in which I sell, the focus is on what will best meet the needs of my clients. I present the most positive image of my offering to be sure, but I don't dismiss as unimportant the alternate solutions available to the client. If I don't listen closely to what my client truly needs or desires and advise him of the best possible solution available to meet these needs, I'm not doing my job correctly. My comparison here is exponentially magnified when one considers that I'm only selling in the commercial realm while the physician deals with critical quality of life issues.

It is here that the cautionary realization should be presented. The medical field is huge business. It operates like few other industries as the profit potential here borders on the incredible. The pressure to sell in the commercial world pales in comparison to the highly competitive medical industry where even the moderately successful are highly compensated and would like to stay that way. Before this experience, I trusted that the physicians primary intent is to give the best medicine. But now I realize that this ideal of trust has become outdated. I was not the only person clinging to the images of the benevolent family doctor, as some recent experiences with other family members' interaction with the medical community have shown me. In one case, the same issues my dad faced with his cancer were faced by another relative.

After I reviewed the sequence of events, I realized that few, if any, options were discussed and the sales cycle for surgery for that family member was completed without a question. He trusted the surgeon. And now this family member is faced with embarrassing complications that he is unprepared to deal with. Complications that have proved detrimental to his quality of life and changed not how we see him, but more importantly, how he sees himself. As a burden.

Perhaps most physicians are honorable people and certainly most are capable of performing the tasks that they advertise. It is the difference in economic realities between now and forty years ago that makes the old image of what doctors used to be now obsolete. Outcome Observations

My final piece of advice is that you be aware of what, in the final analysis, motivates this industry and put strong effort into finding all of the answers that allow options for cure. When choosing a treatment, help your loved one to remain true to who they are. Once you have done that, the paths that are before you become much more easy to navigate. Don't underestimate the value of your support. Taking this journey together is as rewarding for you as it is your loved one.

 # Naturopathic Medicine

Naturopathic Physicians can be identified by the letters N.D. after their names. They are General Practitioners trained as specialists in natural medicine.

Like the more familiar General Practitioners, ND's are educated in conventional medical sciences. However, unlike orthodox MD's, they treat disease and restore health using a wide variety of medical systems: clinical nutrition, homeopathic medicine, botanical medicine, physical medicine, natural childbirth, oriental medicine, counseling and stress management and minor surgery.

They are the only primary care physicians clinically trained in natural therapeutics, tailoring these treatments to the needs of the patient.

With the rise of pharmaceuticals in the 1950's, naturopathic medicine declined in popularity. Health-conscious people looking for non-invasive and less technologically-based treatment at great expense have caused the resurgence of this branch of medicine.

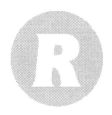

ReSources

Alternative Medicine: The Definitive Guide & Alternative Medicine Yellow Pages
Future Medicine Publishing
1640 Tiburon Blvd. #2
Tiburon, CA 94920.
(800) 333-HEAL

American Association of Naturopathic Physicians (AANP)
2366 Eastlake Avenue East #322
Seattle, WA 98102.
Supports legislation to license and regulate naturopath physicians in all states.
(206) 328-8510.
(206) 323-7610 — referral line.

CANHELP
3111 Paradise Bay Rd.
Port Ludlow, WA 98365.
Information of cancer therapies.
(206) 437-2291.

Cancer Control Society
2043 N. Berendo St.
Los Angeles, CA 90027.
(213) 663-7801.

Dr. Gerald Luna
2520 Longview, Suite 215
Austin, TX 78705. (512) 473-8284.

Exceptional Cancer Patients (Dr. Bernie Siegel's Group)
1302 Chapel St.
New Haven, CT 06511.
(203) 343-5950.

Foundation for the Advancement in Cancer Therapy

Box 1242
Old Chelsea Station
New York, NY 10113.
(212) 741-2790

Healing Choices

C/O Equinox Press
144 St. John Place
Brooklyn, NY. 11217.
Information of cancer therapies.
(718) 636-4433.

International Association of Cancer Victors and Friends

7740 West Manchester Ave. #110
Playa del Rey, CA 90293.
(310) 822-5032.

National Coalition for Cancer Survivorship

1010 Wayne Ave., 5th Floor
Silver Spring, MD 20910.
(301) 650-8868.

Options

by Richard Walters.
Published by Avery Publishing.
Call "People Against Cancer" below.

People Against Cancer

P. O. Box 10, 604 East St.
Otho, IA 50569.
Information of cancer therapies.
(515) 972-4444.

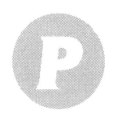

PEPOLE System

How do profiles help us understand an individual and how do we read the profiles? Here is a common profile.:

P	Power	COOPERATIVE	Middle	DOMINANT
E	Extroversion	RESERVED	Middle	OUTGOING
P	Pace	FAST	Middle	PATIENT
O	Organization	CREATIVE	Middle	STRUCTURED
L	Logic	FEELING	Middle	FACT
E	Energy	LITTLE LESS	Same	LOT MORE

I see this about 2 to 3% of the time. Its a "norm line" profile. The individual is not strong or weak on anything.

How about this profile?:

P	Power	COOPERATIVE	Middle	DOMINANT
E	Extroversion	RESERVED	Middle	OUTGOING
P	Pace	FAST	Middle	PATIENT
O	Organization	CREATIVE	Middle	STRUCTURED
L	Logic	FEELING	Middle	FACT
E	Energy	LITTLE LESS	Same	LOT MORE

Ask two questions. If nothing is off to the left, ask which of the four applies the most? "Of these—cooperative, reserved, fast-paced, creative—which applies most to you? Whatever it is, circle

103

it. Then ask of the remaining three (or two, as the case may be), "Which of these—dominant, outgoing, patient, structured—applies most?" Then put in the arrow. So it might look like this:

P	Power	COOPERATIVE	Middle	DOMINANT
E	Extroversion	RESERVED	Middle	OUTGOING
P	Pace	FAST	Middle	PATIENT →
O	Organization	CREATIVE	Middle	STRUCTURED
L	Logic	FEELING	Middle	FACT
E	Energy	LITTLE LESS	Same	LOT MORE

The idea is to force a choice of one of the first four being farthest to the right and one of the first four off to the left. The exception to this is if all four are in the middle.

Okay, this is who I am. That is how you are. What's the best way to get along with you? And what is the best way for you to get along with me?

If a person's trait is farthest to the right or farthest to the left (of the first four), they are:

This is probably more than you need to remember. Just keep in mind the key word—dominant, cooperative, etc. What they circled is what they want. The opposite is what frustrates them.

I strongly encourage you to try it. Do your first "test" with someone who is friendly and believes in you and what you're trying to do: reduce stress in your life. Sometimes this is your life-partner, but not necessarily. As you build up your experience using the System you won't need a card or any kind of copy. You'll just whip out a handy napkin and blaze away. I know you will.

So now we know how to find our perfection. We also know how to find another person's perfection. We know what motivates and frustrates ourselves and others. How do we make it work?

1. Give them what they want. As much as possible, whenever possible, give the other person what they want and do not force

them to do the opposite. If this sounds too simple maybe it is, but this is exactly what happens. Businesses hire dominant people and put them in positions where they have no authority and where they are bossed by an incompetent idiot. In the testing that we have done over the years we find that 80% of those tested were statistically (less than 4.5 on a scale of 10) square pegs in round holes.

Is there any surprise that so many companies have high turnover and absenteeism and low productivity? I'm sure you've seen the bumper sticker "A bad day of fishing is better than a good day of working."

As a boss or manager you can change the situation (and yours and their stress) in five minutes. Do the PEPOLE survey and where possible *unload* those responsibilities that you find are frustrating your workers and give them to those whom the profile shows want them. Example: take the hurry-up duties from the patient worker and give them to the fast-paced one. I'm sure you can see how it works. As far as you can, do it. You will receive an immediate psychological (and spiritual) benefit and the turnover/ productivity figures will start improving the same day.

In your personal life do the same thing. Stop telling Jimmy to hurry up when he's a patient. He'll never hurry up. Praise him for being so patient and persistent. He will love you more and both of your stresses will be reduced. Get the idea? You've got to do the profiles to find out who he is. By the way, people don't have to be able to read these words to make the System work, but they do have to understand them. No understanding = no System. Remember, you only sired these kids, you didn't create them. Its your job to do your best at managing them and their lives.

Wives, lovers, friends, same deal. Give them what they want and praise them for being a perfect whatever they are. They will love you for it, and you will be MUCH more effective in influencing them.

2. Tell them what you want. Denver University did a ten year study on marriage and communication. Couples who took D.U.'s advice and used the new and improved communication style had

half the divorce rate of those in other parts of the country. If you will clearly and repeatedly and lovingly tell people what you want and why, they will give it to you. Example: "I am a patient, deliberate person. Give me the information slowly and *don't* ask me to hurry." Those who don't are then choosing to frustrate you. Get them out of your life.

3. Come together in the middle. I had a partner in a business who was very much the opposite of me. It was in our best interest to work together but it was not in our comfort zone to be like the other. We both knew the PEPOLE System well. When we needed to work and be together, we came to the middle. I was (and am) very fast-paced. He was very patient. When we met I slowed down, he speeded up and for a period of two or three hours we both handled the stress. It was fairly easy because I only had to go to the middle from my fast pace and he only had to go to the middle from his patient pace. It was not easy, but it worked. If I'd had to go to his patient pace or he to my fast pace it would have been very stressful and the relationship would not have worked. This did not mean that he or I had to change (which we really can't do—97% don't change), it meant we had to adjust our behavior during those times that we worked together. This brings us to how do we get along with people we live with, like husbands and wives and kids and such. The obvious answer is to marry the right person in the first place, but most of us don't do that. The problem here gets a little sticky. I'm going to use symbols to show how the solution works. This is over-simplified, but I think you will see how it works. Let's use these symbols to represent different profiles. We're going to define a person as the farthest right or most intense trait. The first four will represent 95% of the population, but we've got some extra symbols so we're including them.

Intense Traits

Dominant		Circle
Outgoing		Triangle
Patient		Square
Structured		Pentagon
Fact Oriented		Hexagon
High Energy		Octagon

What you want in a partner in your business or personal life is not necessarily what you are. We find that in our personal life what we really want in a life partner is:

Almost like ourself   - 25%
Almost the opposite - 25%
A mixture of the two - 50%

So 25% of the time a circle wants a circle and 25% he wants a non-circle and 50% of the time he wants a mixture. Thus a circle may want a triangle, square, pentagon, etc. or he may want a circle. A square might want a square or any other symbol. There is no way I have found of predicting who will want and be successful with whom. Its not what you are that makes you happy but getting what you want. How do you know (or find out) what you want?

Time for a commercial break.

There is a way to find out what you really want in a partner—business or personal. I have a system that will require about five minutes of your time and it will show you what you want. You respond to thirty simple questions. Those responses are put in a computer. A graph and text are generated and Shazaam! The farthest right trait (of the first four) is most important. The second most important is the farthest left. These two together are mostly what you want from a partner. Try it. It works. Its guaranteed. If you aren't satisfied you'll get a refund. The price is $20. Check resources at the end of the book.

End of commercial break.

Finding and keeping a life partner is no easy task. This makes it easier. That's it. That's how the system works.

You give people what they want.

You tell them what you want.

You meet in the middle. I think that's called compromise. The PEPOLE System shows where the middle is.

How about our business life? The System works the same there, except you probably have more people to get along with. Once you have defined your fellow worker's profiles you will be amazed at how much easier it is to get along.

You may find it interesting to test the System. We're all pretty smart about the way we know people, so why not compare what we think BEFORE we do a profile? Why not make your guesses before you ask the six questions? You may be right on all six. I never have nor has anyone else that I've asked. Afterwards, "Oh, yes, I knew he was..." Wrong. You don't know. For years I offered free trips to Paris, Texas, to anyone who could correctly guess another's profile. I haven't had to buy the tickets yet. Here is how to make your guesses: On the left margin of the card, paper, or napkin put arrows to indicate what you think the responses will be. It might look like this.

> if you think the response will be to the right.
< if you think the response will be to the left.
^ if you think the response will be in the middle.

Put a circle around your correct guesses [O] and an [X] through your incorrect ones.

Here's an example of what it might look like:

PEPOLE *Survey   Are you:*

P X	Power	COOPERATIVE	Middle	DOMINANT
E O	Extroversion	RESERVED	Middle	OUTGOING
P O	Pace	FAST	Middle	PATIENT
O X	Organization	CREATIVE	Middle	STRUCTURED
L X	Logic	FEELING	Middle	FACT
E O	Energy	LITTLE LESS	Same	LOT MORE

This person got three out of six, about average. I've seen zero for six and five out of six, but never more.

One of the most stressful parts of any business person's life is hiring, firing, and promoting. When I am hired as a consultant to help companies hire, or do it for them, I use a method that takes only ten minutes and is as close to stress-free as possible. I use a method developed by our company called an occupational profile. It takes us a day or so to do and we give the results free when we do an incentive program for the client. What we do is profile everyone on the job if there are less than twenty people, or only the best ten and the least effective ten if there is a larger total than twenty. We analyze the profiles and come up with a preferred or optimum profile. Variances from that are graded by how far they are from the desired profile and, Whammo! They are given a grade. Data on the candidates physical, mental background and "chemistry" (how much we like each other) is computed and the System develops a highly objective score. The highest scoring candidates are offered the job first. Hiring continues using the remaining applicants until the positions are filled and a "minimum" acceptable scoring level is reached. The system is explained to the applicants and without exception in my experience they like it. Those who are hired are glad they are. To those who do not score well the reasons are explained and they are happy they are not hired for a position for which they are unsuitable. They know it might give them a paycheck but they would be unhappy in the work. A square peg in a round (or triangular, hexagonal, etc.) hole would lead to misery.

So not only are we saving ourselves stress in the hiring process we are saving our clients stress, and certainly the job applicants, too.

Promoting is done the same way. We compare the profiles of the candidates to the "higher" job and promote on the person's compatibility, thus avoiding the "Peter Principle."

As you probably have guessed we have a computer-generated system that gives us more and more accurate information that allows us to make a more valid and more complete assessment of all of the questions we have raised regarding personality profiling and job assessment.

Here is what the questionnaire looks like. We keep it simple so it will be non-threatening. It gives us all the input we need.

PEPOLE PROFILE

DATE:	PHONE:
NAME:	CO:
Enter number for each word. 1 is least, 5 is most.	
How each word describes you	How others would describe you
1. ASSERTIVE	31. COMPETITIVE
2. TALKATIVE	32. LIVELY
3. GENEROUS	33. KIND-HEARTED
4. CONFORMING	34. NICE
5. LOGICAL	35. ACCURATE
6. PRECISE	36. OBJECTIVE
7. LAW-ABIDING	37. TRADITIONAL
8. GOOD-NATURED	38. CALM

PEPOLE PROFILE

9. FRIENDLY	39. CONVINCING
10. DOMINANT	40. CONTROLLING
11. GENTLE	41. RESERVED
12. PRIVATE	42. SILENT
13. DRIVEN	43. IMPATIENT
14. CREATIVE	44. SPONTANEOUS
15. CHARITABLE	45. SYMPATHETIC
16. DETAILED	46. SYSTEMATIC
17. RIGID	47. CONSERVATIVE
18. PERSISTENT	48. PEACEFUL
19. COURAGEOUS	49. PERSUASIVE
20. STRONG-MINDED	50. BOLD
21. INDIVIDUALISTIC	51. DARING
22. OUTGOING	52. CAREFREE
23. RELAXED	53. AGREEABLE
24. RESPECTFUL	54. UNQUESTIONING
25. SENSIBLE	55. ORGANIZED
26. EMOTIONAL	56. CARING
27. INDEPENDENT	57. DISSENTING
28. HURRIED	58. RESTLESS
29. QUIET	59. SERIOUS
30. YIELDING	60. SUBMISSIVE

Don't you need five or ten or fifteen pages of questions to create an accurate instrument? NO. More bulk means more work and more fluff. I am frustrated (stressed) by it and don't have the time and patience for it. I want fast, accurate bottom-line results that tell me what I want to know in as little space as possible. Any-time I try to side-step the System, not only am I wrong, I end up spending hours or weeks to solve the problem I created. My prostate can't afford that anymore. I'm using the System.

There are print-outs available for a number of questions one has in his five lives (Business, Financial, personal, Health and Spiritual) and you are invited to try them all. Every American businessman owes it to himself to do whatever he can reasonably do to reduce his stress and keep his prostate. His company and insurer will probably agree.

Here is what a blank table looks like:

		1	2	3	4	5	6	
POWER	cooperative							dominant
EXTROVERSION	reserved							outgoing
PACE	fast							patient
ORGANIZATION	creative							structured
LOGIC	feel							fact
Energy Style	long							short
Total Energy	efficiency							high
Satisfaction	trust							happy
Stress A								
Stress B								
Stress T								

I committed myself to not doing any people work without using my system. Sometimes it was a temptation to let it go, but I got what I call "crotch throbs" every time I even thought about not staying the course.

To see what a completed one might look like, turn the page.

Here is what a completed chart might look like:

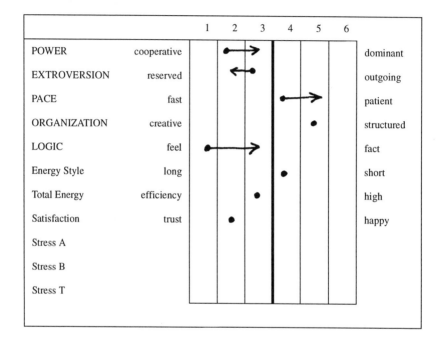

		1	2	3	4	5	6	
POWER	cooperative		•→					dominant
EXTROVERSION	reserved		←•					outgoing
PACE	fast			•→				patient
ORGANIZATION	creative				•			structured
LOGIC	feel	•→						fact
Energy Style	long			•				short
Total Energy	efficiency		•					high
Satisfaction	trust	•						happy
Stress A								
Stress B								
Stress T								

New Treatments

Channel 13 News in Houston, Texas, reported that Dr. James Herman at Baylor College of Medicine—Prostate Diagnostic Center was injecting cancer tumors with a common cold rhinovirus. In tests of ten individuals, this treatment has appeared to effectively eliminate the cancer. Further FDA tests are being scheduled for ten other individuals at a higher level of virus dosage with more impressive results expected.

A 1995 study from Harvard School of Public Health found that men who ate tomato products were 45% less likely to develop prostate cancer than men who ate small amounts of those foods. Why? An anti-oxidant lycopene tends to accumulate in the prostate and may help block the start of the disease. Some 47,000 men were questioned about their dietary habits for this study.

Cooper Clinic in Dallas announced results of their study which showed that exercise was associated with much lower rates of prostate cancer. There were 13,000 subjects in this study. A 1992 Harvard Alumni Health Study showed that men over 70 using heavy exercise (4,000 calories a week in physical activities) encountered only half the prostate cancer as those who did not burn as many calories.

High fat diets have a link to prostate cancer, says the American Cancer Society.

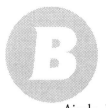

Bibliography

Airola, Paavo O. Ph.D., N.D. *Cancer: Causes, Prevention and Treatment—The Total Approach* and *How To Get Well*. Phoenix, AZ: Health Plus, 1972 and 1974.

Bethel, May. The Healing Power of Herbs. Wilshire, CA: Wilshire Book Co., 1995.

Bieler, Henry G., M.D., and Maxine Block. *Food Is YOur Best Medicine*. New York: Ballantine Books, 1987.

Brennan, Richard O., M.D., and Helen K. Hosier. Coronary? *Cancer? God's Answer: Prevent It!* Irvine, CA: Harvest House Publishers, 1979.

"Cancer and Diet, An East West Foundation Publication," Brookline, MA: East West Foundation, 1980.

Clark, Hulga Regehr , Ph.D., ND. *The Cure For All Cancer*. San Diego, CA: Promotion Publishing, 1995.

Cousins, Norman. *Anatomy of an Illness as Perceived by the Patient.* New York: Bantam Books, 1983.

Donsbach, Kurt W., Ph.D., D.Sc., N.D., D.C. *Metabolic Cancer Therapies*. Huntington Beach, CA: The International Institute of Natural Health Sciences, Inc., 1981.

Fink, John M. *Third Opinion: An International Directory to Alternative Therapy Centers for Treatment and Prevention of Cancer.* Wayne, NJ: Avery Publishing, Inc., 1988.

Fischer, William. *How to Fight Cancer and Win*. Canfield, OH: Fischer Publishing, 1987.

Frähm, Anne E., and David J. Frähm. *A Cancer Battle Plan: Six Strategies for Beating Cancer from a Recovered Hopeless Case.* Colorado Springs, CO: Piñon Press, 1992.

Gerson, Max, M.D. *A Cancer Therapy: Results of Fifty Cases.* Bonita, CA :The Gerson Institute, 1990.

Harper, Harowd, M.D., and Michael Culbert. *How You Can Beat the Killer Diseases.* New Rochelle, NY: Arlington House, 1977.

Holmes, Marjorie. *God and Vitamins.* New York: Avon Books, 1980.

Hunsberger, Eydie Maye, and Chris Loeffler. *How I Conquered Cancer Naturally.* Eugene, OR: Harvest House Publishers, 1975.

McCabe, John. *Surgery Electives: What To Know Before The Doctor Operates.* Santa Monica, CA: Carmania Books, 1997.

Quillin, Patrick, Ph.D., R.D. *Healing Nutrients.* New York: Random House, 1989.

Robbins, John. *Diet for a New America.* Walpole, NH: Stillpoint Publishing, 1987.

Salaman, Maureen, M.Sc. *Nutrition: The Cancer Answer.* Statford, CA: Statford Publishing, 1984.

Siegel, Bernie, M.D. *Love, Medicine and Miracles.* New York: Harper & Row, 1988.

Simon, Charles B., M.D. *Cancer and Nutrition.* New York: McGraw-Hill, 1983.

Simonton, Carl, M.D., Stephanie Matthews-Simonton, and James Creighton. *Getting Well Again.* Los Angeles, CA: J. P. Tarcher, Inc., 1978.

Smythe, Benjamin Roth. *Killing Cancer: The Jason Winters Story.* Las Vegas, NV: Vinton Publishing, 1980.

Stiewing, Patti. *Embrace The Angel.* Nashville, TN: Tobias & Co., 1996.

Twoner, Bettie. *Cancer Holiday.* Seattle, WA: Greenlake Publishers, 1978.

Vonderplanitz, Aajonus. *We Want To Live. Volume I: Out of the Grips of Disease and Death* and *Volume II: Healthfully.* Los Angeles, CA: Carnelian Bay Castle Press, 1996.

Weil, Andrew. *Spontaneous Healing: How to Discover and Enhance Your Body's Natural Ability to Maintain and Heal Itself.* New York: Alfred A. Knopf, 1995.

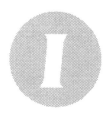

Index

PRODUCTS YOU'LL FIND HELPFUL
FROM THE AUTHOR OF
HOW I CONQUERED CANCER

How I Conquered Cancer

Includes his personal story, a useful bibliography, resources, addresses and phone numbers for more information.

Additional copies	$9.95
5 or more copies (each)	$7.95
Even more copies	Quote

The Velvet Glove

The first of Eric Gardiner's books, this volume shows how to use personality profiling to communicate clearly with business and social partners. Carl Victor Hansen contributed the Foreword. He loved it!

Single copies	$9.95
Multiple copies	Quote

PEPOLE Personality Profiles $20.00

Get a sample FREE — one per customer, please. A small processing & handling fee is only $3.

Partner Preference Profile $20.00

Get a sample FREE — one per customer, please. A small processing & handling fee is only $3.

Occupational Profiles $200.00

For each job description

Get a sample FREE for qualified prospects who do hiring or stress seminars— one per customer, please. A small procssing and handling fee is only $50.

Seminars

Hiring, promotion, partner profile	Free! Pay expenses only.
Family, relationships, dating, marriage	Free!
Pay expenses only.	
Cancer and how I conquered it	Free!
Pay expenses only.	
Stress measurement and reduction	
(company or personal level)	Free!
Pay expenses only.	

CALL (800) 324-5662
TO
SCHEDULE AND CO-ORDINATE SEMINARS.